Japanese Hot Stone Massage

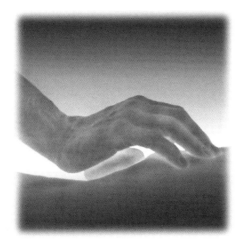

Mark Hess & Shogo Mochizuki

Japanese Hot Stone Massage

Published in the United States by

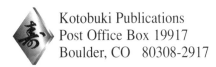

Kotobuki Publications
Post Office Box 19917
Boulder, CO   80308-2917

ISBN : 1-57615-150-6

Library of Congress Cataloging-in-Publication Data

Printed in the United States
First Edition

japanese hot stone massage v. 1.1-D   05-15-02

Acknowledgements

We have many people to thank for their help in the process of creating this book. This book would not have been possible without each person's unique contributions, both direct and indirect. We appreciate their support, and it is our hope that the readers of this book see the value of their contributions and positive energy.

Special Thank You to the following people:
- Jaime Schwalb — Editor
- Takahito Gomi — Cover design, Photo Adjustments
- Peggy Kennedy Thomason — Illustrations
- Michael Keefe — Photographer
- Jay Kinghorn — Photographer
- Shinji Tsuji — Photographer
- Mayo Furuya — Model
- Jane Sears — Model
- Diane Washburn — Model

Thanks to many of our friends who have supported this project in numerous ways.

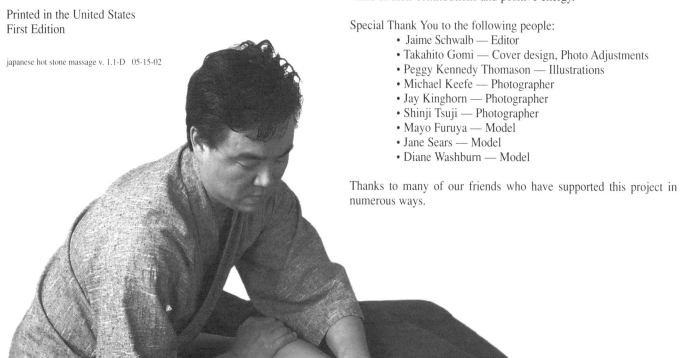

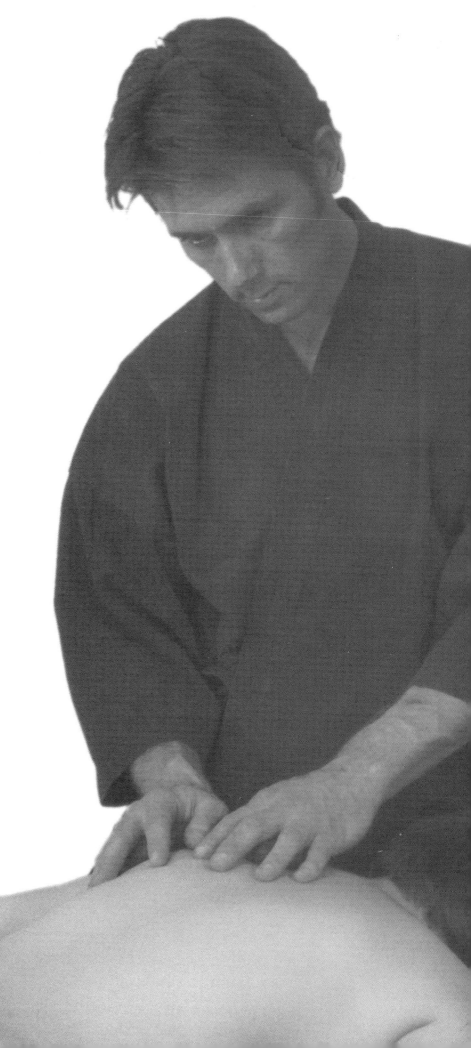

温石按摩

Japanese
Hot Stone
Massage

Japanese Hot

table of contents

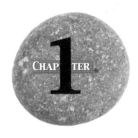
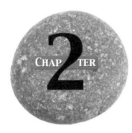
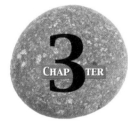

Stone Massage

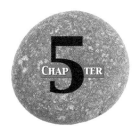
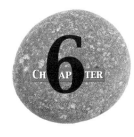
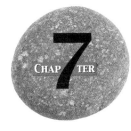

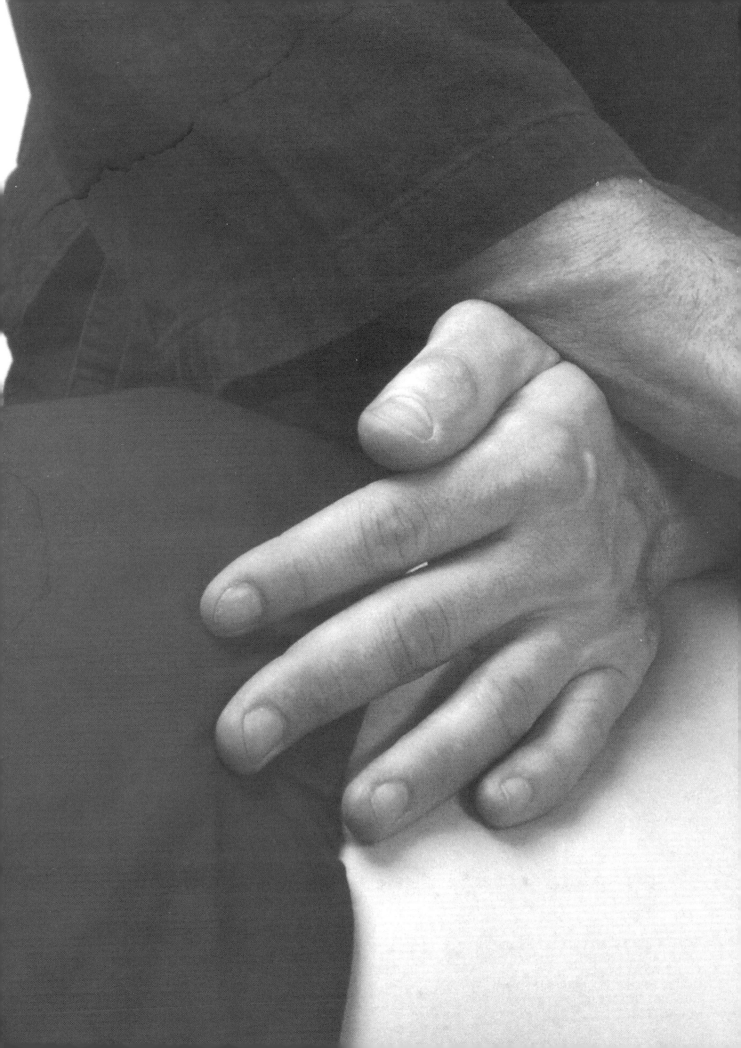

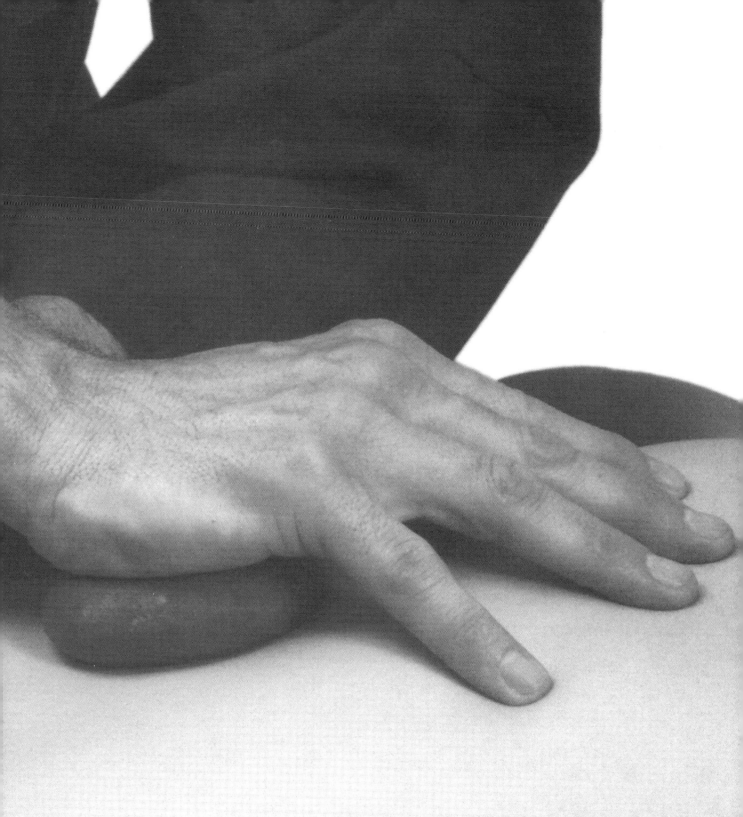

Chapter One
ANCIENT WISDOM

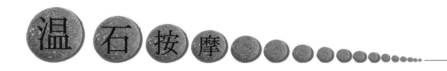

Chapter One
ANCIENT WISDOM

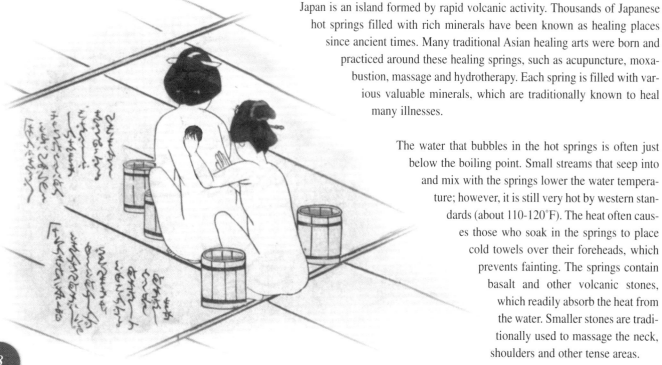

Japan is an island formed by rapid volcanic activity. Thousands of Japanese hot springs filled with rich minerals have been known as healing places since ancient times. Many traditional Asian healing arts were born and practiced around these healing springs, such as acupuncture, moxabustion, massage and hydrotherapy. Each spring is filled with various valuable minerals, which are traditionally known to heal many illnesses.

The water that bubbles in the hot springs is often just below the boiling point. Small streams that seep into and mix with the springs lower the water temperature; however, it is still very hot by western standards (about 110-120°F). The heat often causes those who soak in the springs to place cold towels over their foreheads, which prevents fainting. The springs contain basalt and other volcanic stones, which readily absorb the heat from the water. Smaller stones are traditionally used to massage the neck, shoulders and other tense areas.

Japanese Hot Stone Massage evolves from these ancient hot spring traditions to introduce the same therapeutic value into modern therapy environments.

Massage originated from the human instinct to rub and apply pressure in order to alleviate aches and pains. Over many years of experimentation, healers learned that manipulating specific areas was most effective in promoting good health. It was also discovered that massaging with heated stones was an effective and efficient way to heal and reduce muscle tension.

Japanese Hot Stone Massage is based upon anma, the oldest form of East Asian massage. Anma is rooted in ancient Nepal, Tibet and western China, where it was developed over 7,000 years ago. Anma entered Japan along with traditional medicine, such as acupuncture and herbal medicine, over 1,300 years ago. Anma is a kneading, rotation and vibration-based massage. It is intricately woven into the tapestry of Japanese history and culture and is a deeply respected art form. Unlike newer therapies created within the last century, anma has undergone thousands of years of refinement. It is no longer in a developmental stage, but exists as a very stable, perfected form.

Although acupuncture dates back 7,000 years, needle insertion did not begin until 2,000 years ago. Before that, stones were often used to stimulate acupoints and meridians in order to restore balance in the human body. Moxabustion consists of applying heat into tsubo points and is always applied with acupuncture, with which it shares many historical links. Japanese Hot Stone Massage creates similar effects to moxabustion, because the warmth from the stones also stimulates tsubo points. Stones can stimulate tsubo points, allowing heat to penetrate the point, like moxabustion. However, all traditional Japanese massage teaching dictates that massage techniques be applied before stimulating tsubo points. Therefore, Japanese Hot Stone Massage is not simply a massage with hot stones, it combines acupuncture, moxabustion and massage for a complete and therapeutic treatment.

Ancient traditions preserve essential beliefs which encourage the culture's evolution along pathways, marked and shepherded by principles of wisdom. When we study an ancient tradition, we are exposed to its richness, which unfolds in a way that accommodates the learning experience, while being nurtured by the past. It is a delight to experience the realm of traditional training, because we acquire knowledge by following the path that has led centuries of students to succeed. There is great respect for the traditional arts in Japan. Any traditional art takes significant time to master, but when this time is invested, one learns the art in a genuine way.

Japanese Hot Stone Massage is one of the most powerful, therapeutic treatments and we introduce it to the Western world, not only as a form of massage, but as traditional art and ancient wisdom.

Benefits of Japanese Hot Stone Massage

- Japanese Hot Stone Massage relieves stress caused by modern lifestyles and occupations by balancing the *ki* (body energy) to restore and improve health.

- This style of massage can be gentle and calm to relieve stress, or deep and penetrating to reduce significant back, neck and shoulder tension; therefore, it is well-suited for any type of spa or private practice environment.

- Techniques introduced in this book are easy to learn and do not require previous hot stone massage training, so you can use them immediately and improve your treatment today.

- Japanese Hot Stone Massage can be performed without prior knowledge of Asian bodywork concepts, such as *yin/yang* and five element theory; however, a deeper understanding of those theories will enhance your skills.

- You can quickly adapt these techniques into your existing hot stone massage practice to enhance your repertoire and offer your clients a new, exciting treatment.

- Japanese Hot Stone treatments are the only non-oil hot stone modalities and can be applied over draping to accommodate clients who have allergic reactions or are sensitive to oils or lotions. It is also well-suited for circumstances when the client must remain fully draped.

- These techniques can be seamlessly integrated into non-oil modalities, such as shiatsu and Asian bodywork.

- You can also apply these techniques with lubrication to seamlessly adapt them into your swedish, deep tissue or other lubrication based practice.

- If you have thumb and hand injuries or your hands easily fatigue, Japanese Hot Stone Massage is excellent, because it creates very little stress on your hands.

- Japanese Hot Stone Massage requires less body movement than any other form of hot stone massage, except Shiatsu with Hot Stones. Therefore, it minimizes therapist effort during treatments, which will potentially increase the number of treatments you can perform in one day.

- This book teaches proper and improper body mechanics, so you will learn how to to minimize stress to your body during treatments. As you study Japanese Hot Stone Massage, you will naturally adapt better body mechanics into your practice.

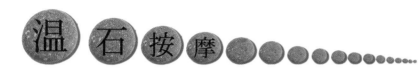

History of Traditional Japanese Massage

Anma (Anmo, in Chinese pronunciation), traditional Japanese massage, and East Asian medicine date back to prehistoric times, as much as 4,000 to 10,000 years ago. Throughout the proto-historic period (2783–1123 B.C.E.), different components of East Asian medicine originated in multiple places. In eastern China, surgical instruments were being produced, while in the central region, *do in* and *an kyo* were developed to stretch and massage the muscles. Much of anma is thought to have developed in central China; however, literature found in Japan indicates that anma may have originated in regions of Nepal, Tibet and northern India.

During the Zhou and Qin Dynasties (1122–207 B.C.E.), all of the regional medical practices were tested and systemized to determine their medical viability. The *Su Wen* and *Ling Shu* were also written during this period. These texts detail pathological concepts and East Asian medical treatments. This is the first time that anma was recorded in literature that included information about techniques and treatment methods.

During the early and late Han Dynasties (221 B.C.E.–C.E. 264), Emperor Huang Ti spearheaded the creation of the *Huang Ti Nei Ching, The Yellow Emperor's Classic of Internal Medicine*. A system of schooling in traditional Chinese medicine was established during this time, based upon the *Huang Ti Nei Ching*. This system consisted of seven schools and 216 texts for acupuncture, eleven schools and 274 texts for herbal medicine, eight schools and 186 texts concerning sexual practices, and ten schools and 205 texts on remedial exercises, such as *do-in*. Only eighteen volumes of the *Yellow Emperor's Classic of Internal Medicine* remain. Those eighteen volumes are the oldest existing medical texts in the world.

Anma was introduced to Japan from China, through Korea in the early part of the fifth century. From the early fifth century to the Asuka Period (C.E. 710), Japan actively traded with China through Korea and the basis for modern Japanese culture was formed. In C.E. 562, Chi So, a Chinese monk/physician, brought 160 Chinese medical texts (including acupuncture) to Japan and became a Japanese citizen. During the Nara and Heian Periods (C.E. 710–1185), Japan began formalizing more of its medical education system. In C.E. 718, the Japanese government established a medical school for the systematic study of acupuncture and other healing modalities. An anma degree or a degree as a medical incantation therapist (*ju gon shi*) required three years of study. Although acupuncture's history dates back more than 5,000 years, needle insertion did not actually begin until about 2,000 years ago. Before needle insertion, sharp stones and other metal objects were pressed against the skin to stimulate tsubo. During an excavation, Japanese archeologists discovered sharp stone (flint) needles that date back to the 5th Century C.E., which were most likely used to externally stimulate tsubo.

In C.E. 753, a Chinese Buddhist monk named Jiang Zhen emigrated to Japan with thirty-five doctors who served as his disciples and transmitted their knowledge to Japanese monks and students. In C.E. 984, thirteen volumes of *I Shin Bo*, the oldest medical text in Japan, were published by Yasuyori Tanba by commission of the Emperor. The *I Shin Bo* covered all known medical subjects, including anma, acupuncture, moxabustion and 658 tsubo. During the turbulent Kamakura and Muromachi Periods (C.E. 1185–1574), support for the official medical system was abandoned and Japanese medicine began to decline. The common people, however, continued practicing anma, acupuncture and moxabustion.

Japanese medical development began to flourish again during the Momoyama Period (C.E. 1575–1602). During this time, the capital was moved from western Japan to the east (near Yokohama and across from Tokyo), and there were many new developments in anma. In 1602, when Edo (Tokyo) became the capital city, Japanese medicine and bodywork began to develop even more. Many new techniques were developed in both acupuncture and anma. These techniques were recorded in a new series of texts and taught in new schools that were established in Tokyo.

During the Edo Period (C.E. 1602–1868), Western medical knowledge was introduced to Japan for the first time by physicians who accompanied the Dutch Trading Company. The Dutch physicians were also exposed to Japanese medical knowledge, including anma and acupuncture, which they soon brought back to Europe.

During the Meiji Period (C.E. 1868–1912), the shoguns lost power and there was a rise of imperialistic politics in Japan. The Japanese government was then modeled after the Western model, which westernized Japanese society. Western medicine replaced traditional Asian medicine as the primary method of treatment, nearly wiping out the traditional therapeutic use of anma and East Asian medicine.

In the early 1900's, a new therapy called shiatsu was developed by Tokojiro Namikoshi and other therapists; however, it was still categorized as a part of anma. Then, in 1964, the government developed guidelines and licensing procedures, making shiatsu a modality independent from anma.

The industrialization of Japan led to many changes in the lifestyles of its citizens, and anma has adapted to accommodate those changes. Changes in the work style meant longer hours, different types of labor and increased stress in daily life. Many advanced therapists reintroduced the concepts of *keiraku* and tsubo in order to address the increasing number of ailments from job-related stress and changes in employment conditions. Anma has survived and flourished for centuries by evolving and changing to accommodate the needs of modern life, while retaining its ancient therapeutic and healing value.

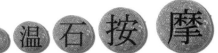

Traditional Japanese View of Health

Japanese and Western philosophies about health are culturally distinct. Understanding the traditional Japanese perspective on health care will optimize your understanding of Japanese Hot Stone Massage.

In the West, people tend not to recognize illness until they have been diagnosed by a physician, and treatment does not usually begin until they suffer from severe symptoms. Little effort is usually made to strengthen the body before disease sets in. In Japan, treatment takes place much earlier. Traditional Japanese medical providers detect illness in the early diagnostic stages and instruct their patients to take preventative measures. When noticeable symptoms appear, the illness is considered advanced. Once treatment begins, it usually takes as long to rebalance the body as it took for the imbalance to occur.

Traditional Japanese culture values and respects longevity, with the idea that through "harmonizing heaven and earth" (that is to say, balancing the mind and body), one can attain a long life with minimal difficulties. In traditional Japanese medicine, practitioners help guide clients back into harmony with nature. They do not merely relieve pain, they restore harmony between heaven and earth, so patients may live out their full life span.

In East Asia, many people trust ancient medicine, because it is rich in historical and cultural tradition. Except for subtle additions and modifications, many Japanese and Chinese health care practices have remained relatively unchanged for 2,000 years. In the United States, there are few traditional healing methods based on time-tested remedies, and alternative medicine is often viewed with suspicion. The medicine practiced today in the West is extremely different from medicine practiced just fifty years ago. The sense of cultural tradition, heritage and continuity found in the East is not as strong in Western medical practices. Western and Eastern medicine play very different roles within their respective cultures.

Western culture fosters a static ideal of perfect health, as if it were something one could attain at once, then maintain through exercise and diet. Most Westerners want an instant cure and are not always willing to take steps to gradually improve their health. Most East Asians, on the other hand, do not believe in "perfect" health, because health is always shifting in and out of balance. Constantly striving for balance is the objective, and achieving balance is the goal.

Mainstream Western health care generally treats only the symptoms, while East Asian disciplines dictate that one must balance the entire body in order to effectively treat a single affliction. East Asian disciplines use a truly holistic approach—organ systems, muscular systems and circulatory systems, along with emotional, psychological and spiritual health, are all considered to be interdependent factors.

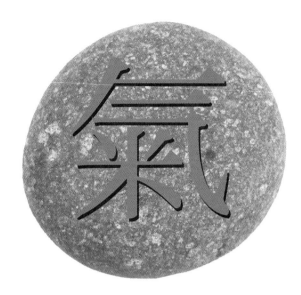

Ki

Ki, or *qi* as the Chinese pronounce it, is becoming a familiar word in the Western world; however, it is difficult to precisely define *ki*. Westerners often translate *ki* as "energy," but this translation is inadequate. In reality, the concept of *ki* embraces every aspect of human life.

In Japan, *ki* is intricately connected to daily life. For example, people ask, "How is your *ki* today?" instead of "How are you?" and disease is described as a *ki* illness (*byo ki*). In the West, there is no identical concept of an integrated sense of being, such as *ki*. In our experience, Westerners often have great difficulty understanding *ki*, because it cannot be explained intellectually.

According to traditional Taoist theory, there are three different types of *ki* energy that affect everything in the universe: *ten ki*, *ji ki*, and *jin ki*. In dealing with human health, healing arts practitioners generally only deal with *jin ki*, the human *ki* energy. Human *ki* energy is, however, so affected by heaven *ki* and earth *ki*, that total wellness depends upon the balance between all three energies. In fact, heaven *ki*, which is air, and earth *ki*, which is food and water, combine to create the primary function of human *ki* energy. In other respects, all living creatures require the same combination of heaven *ki* and earth *ki* to survive. Both the condition of air and the quality of food and water affect the human body's ability to function. When the quality and quantity of heaven *ki* and earth *ki* are insufficient, human *ki* becomes prone to illness. For example, if a person lives in a large city, eats a diet of fast food, breathes low quality air and is under heavy stress, the quality of his *ki* will be diminished and his health will greatly suffer. Heaven *ki* and earth *ki* do not seem closely connected during treatment, but they become essential for determining the cause of many illnesses.

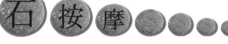

Yin/Yang and Five Elements Theories

Most people recognize the symbol of *yin/yang*. The concept of *yin/yang* is about "balance" between opposites. *Yin* and *yang* is the Chinese pronunciation for this concept, but in Japanese, it's pronounced *in* and *yo*. This concept is essential for understanding and practicing anma, as well as traditional East Asian medicine. Traditional East Asian medicine is all about balance—the more balanced a person is, the healthier they are.

All traditional Japanese medicine is based upon the Taoist concepts of opposites (*Yin/Yang* Theory) and is a part of five categories or elements, which is known as the Five Elements Theory. The theories of *Yin/Yang* and the Five Elements developed at separate times and places. It is commonly understood that *Yin/Yang* Theory is much older and was developed first. In Five Elements Theory, everything in the universe is placed into one of five categories: Fire, Earth (Soil), Metal, Water and Wood. As in *Yin/Yang* Theory, it is most important to keep everything balanced and in harmony.

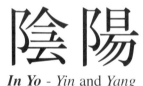

In Yo - *Yin* and *Yang*

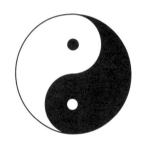

Yin/Yang Symbol

In traditional East Asian medical theory, *yin* is often considered more important than *yang*, because the purpose of *yang* is to support *yin*. The main function of the *yang* organs is to support the *yin* organs of the same element; likewise, the main function of the *yang* meridians is to support the functions of the *yin* meridians of the same element. There is no absolute *yin* or *yang*, this is why each contains a portion of the other. A black circle inside the white and a white circle inside the black illustrate that all *yin* contains some *yang* and vice versa. For example, absolute darkness (*yin*) does not exist, nor does absolute brightness (*yang*). All darkness contains some brightness, just as all brightness contains some darkness.

A common misunderstanding about *Yin/Yang* theory is that *yang* is good and *yin* is bad. In truth, neither is better or worse than the other; both are equally important aspects of the whole. Without understanding negative, one cannot understand positive and without understanding the female, one cannot understand the male. Two opposite aspects must be balanced in *yin* and *yang* to function properly, because they drive each other. *Yin/Yang* philosophy is not about making a judgement of better or worse, but about achieving balance.

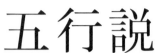

Go Gyo Setsu
Five Elements Theory

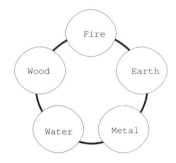

In Five Elements Theory, everything—time, seasons, directions, animals, planets, smells and internal organs—belongs to one of five categories. The combination of *Yin/Yang* and Five Elements theories comprises the foundation of Japanese acupuncture and bodywork, and can be traced back to the Zhou Dynasty (1122 B.C.E.). These theories entered Japan in the fifth century and are the distinct properties of Japanese bodywork and acupuncture.

The mutual or beginning position of the five elements is shown above and on the opposite page. This shows the five elements maintaining a harmonious, balanced, mutual relationship. This position represents perfect balance in nature and internal organ balance in Japanese medicine—no single part interferes with another—and indicates perfectly balanced physical and psychological health. Such placement and balance is the ideal state.

The creative cycle, also called the Mother-Son Law, represents the natural phenomenon of regeneration or creation, when one element creates the next element. An essential relationship exists between the creating and created elements. For example, Water is necessary for the creation of Wood, and Wood is necessary for the creation of Fire. If an element is depleted, the creating element needs support in order to tonify the element that needs to be created.

The destructive cycle represents the natural phenomenon of destruction or control of one element over another. One element can be a destroyer and another element can be destroyed. For instance, Water in excess can destroy Fire, which is recognized as the destroyer controlling the destroyed element.

温石按摩

The combination of *Yin/Yang* and Five Elements theories shown here is commonly used in traditional Japanese and East Asian medicine. Ten internal organs are placed in relationships between *yin* and *yang* and among the five elements.

Anma works within these theories to equally distribute *ki* throughout the ten internal organs. It can be very complex to address all ten internal organs at once. It is more effective and less complex to first balance the *yin* and *yang* in each individual element, then create balance among the five elements.

These relationships illustrate the balance of the internal organs, which is the ideal sought by those who practice anma, traditional Japanese and East Asian medicine. Understanding how these organs interrelate is critical when practicing any East Asian healing art.

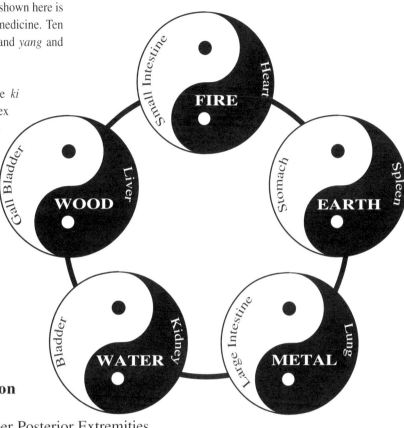

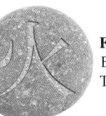

Fire Element: Passion
Emotion: Joy
Techniques for the Upper Posterior Extremities

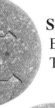

Soil Element: Rejuvenation
Emotion: Worry
Techniques for the Lower Posterior Extremities

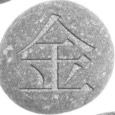

Metal Element: Balancing
Emotion: Sadness
Techniques for the Upper Anterior Extremities

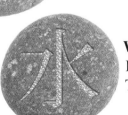

Water Element: Calming
Emotion: Fear
Techniques for the Anterior Lower Extremities

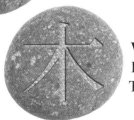

Wood Element: Transformation
Emotion: Anger
Techniques for Finishing the Treatment

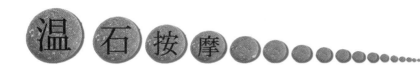
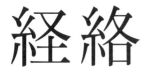

経絡

Meridians

Keiraku, commonly translated as "Meridian System," is the channel or pathway system for *ki* energy. *Keiraku* is traditionally used in Japanese massage, because it evolved with other forms of East Asian medicine. *Keiraku* is a liquid vessel with a diameter of twenty to fifty-five millimicrons. It is the pathway for a clear, transparent liquid (*toeki*) and works much like a nerve.

The *keiraku* (*ching-lo* in Chinese) system consists of 100 meridians and their connections. The *keiraku* is both a *kei* system and a *raku* system. The *kei* system consists of thirty-two meridian vessels: twelve standard *kei* meridians connected from internal organs, twelve branch meridians and eight vessels. The remaining sixty-eight vessels compose the *raku* system and its connections.

The twelve standard *kei* meridians are:

1)	*Hai kei*	Lung Meridian
2)	*Dai cho kei*	Large Intestine Meridian
3)	*I kei*	Stomach Meridian
4)	*Hi kei*	Spleen Meridian
5)	*Shin kei*	Heart Meridian
6)	*Sho cho kei*	Small Intestine Meridian
7)	*Bo ko kei*	Bladder Meridian
8)	*Jin kei*	Kidney Meridian
9)	*Shin po kei*	*Shin Po* Meridian
10)	*San sho kei*	*San Sho* Meridian
11)	*Tan kei*	Gall Bladder Meridian
12)	*Kan kei*	Liver Meridian

The twelve *kei* meridians are connected to each other in the order listed above, and they form two bilaterally symmetric loops on either side of the body. It takes exactly twenty-four hours for *ki* to cycle through these twelve meridians.

The eight vessels divide the body into different sectors to balance the meridians. The two vessels that travel along the median line (center line) on the front and the back are the two vessels most often used for treatment.

13)	*Nin myaku*	Conception vessel
14)	*Toku myaku*	Governing vessel

The combination of two these vessels and the twelve standard *kei* meridians is commonly called the "fourteen meridians of the body." These fourteen meridians are primarily used for diagnosis and treatment in East Asian medicine.

Tsubo

When we feel aches or pains, our natural response is to touch the painful area to find the exact source of the pain. Applying simple pressure or rubbing these points often eases the pain. The conceptualization of tsubo occurred over 3,000 years ago in China in response to the discovery that certain painful points on the body were common to all people. Since that time, tsubo has become systematized and well-developed. It forms the foundation for traditional Chinese and Japanese medicine and anma.

Tsubo is often translated as "acupoint" or "acupuncture point." In our teaching and in this book, we refer to these points as tsubo. Tsubo are points on the body that can be stimulated in order to relieve pain, or to produce certain effects on the internal organs and relieve symptoms.
    Using tsubo and *keiraku* can be effective in anma treatments.

The character for tsubo originated in China at least 3,000 years ago. It is a Chinese hieroglyph that literally translates as "jar." On the body, a tsubo is shaped like a tiny jar or deep pore.

One important concept of traditional East Asian medicine is to imagine things in the universe that are invisible to the eye, like air. Imagine the tsubo as a small jar right beneath the skin, which is filled with stagnant *ki*. Your fingertips are like lids, but they also have the power to go into the tsubo and rejuvenate the stagnating *ki*.

Tsubo is the most important concept for the effective use of anma during a treatment. Applying pressure to the appropriate tsubo in anma and shiatsu ensures the release of stagnating *ki*. To understand stagnant *ki*, it is helpful to visualize a meridian as a hose with water running through it. The liquid (*toeki*) carries *ki* through the body. A tsubo is a point where stagnation commonly occurs on the meridian, just as kinks prevent water from flowing freely through a hose.

There are two categories of tsubo: *kei ketsu*, which are located on top of twelve meridians and two vessels, and *ki ketsu*, which are not located on the meridians (there are about 750 on each side of the body). The study of tsubo focuses mainly on *kei ketsu*. There are approximately 361 *kei ketsu* tsubo on each side of the body. They can be thought of as a stagnation or counterpoint of the meridian.

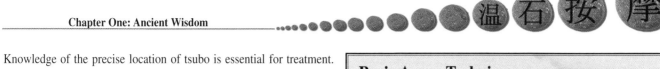

Knowledge of the precise location of tsubo is essential for treatment. Some tsubo are smaller than others, and if the practitioner is off by even one-sixteenth of an inch, effective treatment is impossible. Tsubo are generally located near the tip of a nerve or at a weak spot on the body, such as between the muscles and bones. Tsubo are normally located in slight depressions or indentations on the body. Through physical examination, these depressions can help you identify the exact location of a tsubo. The best way to learn the location of tsubo points is to try and identify them on your own body. This way, you can feel the different sensations of pain and pressure at each point, while learning their precise location.

Pain at a particular tsubo is often an indication of some irregularity in the physical and/or internal organs. Slightly different symptoms occur in each individual, because each body is unique. The response to tsubo stimulation varies as well.

Tsubo, meridians and all concepts of East Asian medicine require intensive study to fully understand and perform. One must first be able to diagnose conditions using pulse or abdominal diagnosis—an essential part of traditional East Asian medical treatment. One must also have a deep understanding of East Asian medical theory, meridians and tsubo. Basic knowledge of western anatomy, physiology and pathology is helpful, but unnecessary. In-depth study of meridians and tsubo in traditional East Asian medicine can often take several years.

Out of 361 points of tsubo, most acupuncturists and East Asian body-workers use 130 to 200 for an individual treatment. Other points are used for less common circumstances, but it is very rare for practitioners to use every tsubo point in one treatment. Certain tsubo are commonly used to treat an array of illnesses, while other points are rarely used for only very obscure conditions.

This book explains meridians and a few of their tsubo as an introduction, but the primary focus is on the basic techniques that are at the heart of anma. Proper understanding of Japanese Hot Stone Massage techniques is the basic requirement for performing an effective treatment. Treatments using meridians and tsubo can enhance a practitioner's massage, but only after the primary techniques are well developed. You will still be able to give an excellent massage without a deep understanding of meridians and tsubo.

Basic Anma Techniques

Japanese Hot Stone Massage is based on techniques from anma, traditional Japanese massage. Anma contains seven categories of techniques:

- **Light Stroking Technique** (*Kei Satsu Ho*) is performed by sliding over the body surface with either up and down or circular motions. Light stroking is used to gently warm the surface area, relax the muscles and improve circulation.

- **Kneading Technique** (*Ju Netsu Ho*) is the primary anma technique. Kneading is usually applied by engaging the underlying tissue in a rotating or kneading movement to effectively reduce muscle tension. This technique does not slide over the skin or fabric and should be applied after warming the area.

- **Vibration Technique** (*Shin Sen Ho*), a frequently used anma technique, is often used to disperse the intensity of pressure when treating a sensitive region. Vigorous shaking also helps move toxins into the blood or lymphatic systems.

- **Pressure Technique** (*Ap Paku Ho*) was once the primary anma technique. From the early 20th century, people who specialized in pressure techniques were known as shiatsu therapists. Shiatsu later became an independent therapy. This pressure technique compresses the muscle to release tension, and stimulates tsubo to restore balance in the human body.

- **Percussion Technique** (*Ko Da Ho*) is a fast, gentle tapping technique, not a hitting technique. This technique is generally applied toward the end of treatment to disperse toxins into the blood and lymphatic systems. This technique is not well-suited for hot stone massage.

- **Special Percussion Technique** (*Kyoku Te Ho*) requires you to change the shape of your hand when applying percussion. This technique is not applicable for hot stone massage, because you cannot change the shape of your hands while holding stones.

- **Stretching and Movement Technique** (*Un Do Ho*) is a series of stretching and movement techniques. It can be used on its own, but it is generally combined with other techniques, such as applying pressure while moving the arms or legs.

Understanding the Symbols in This Book

To accompany the written explanation, we have placed different arrows over the pictures to visually explain different types of movement.

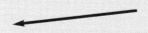

A bold arrow indicates that the stone is sliding over the surface of the skin. This technique is a light stroking technique.

A dotted arrow indicates that you manipulate the muscle or engage the underlying tissue, while moving within the elasticity of the skin. The stone does not slide over the skin.

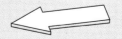

Three dimensional arrows indicate the direction of body movement or application.

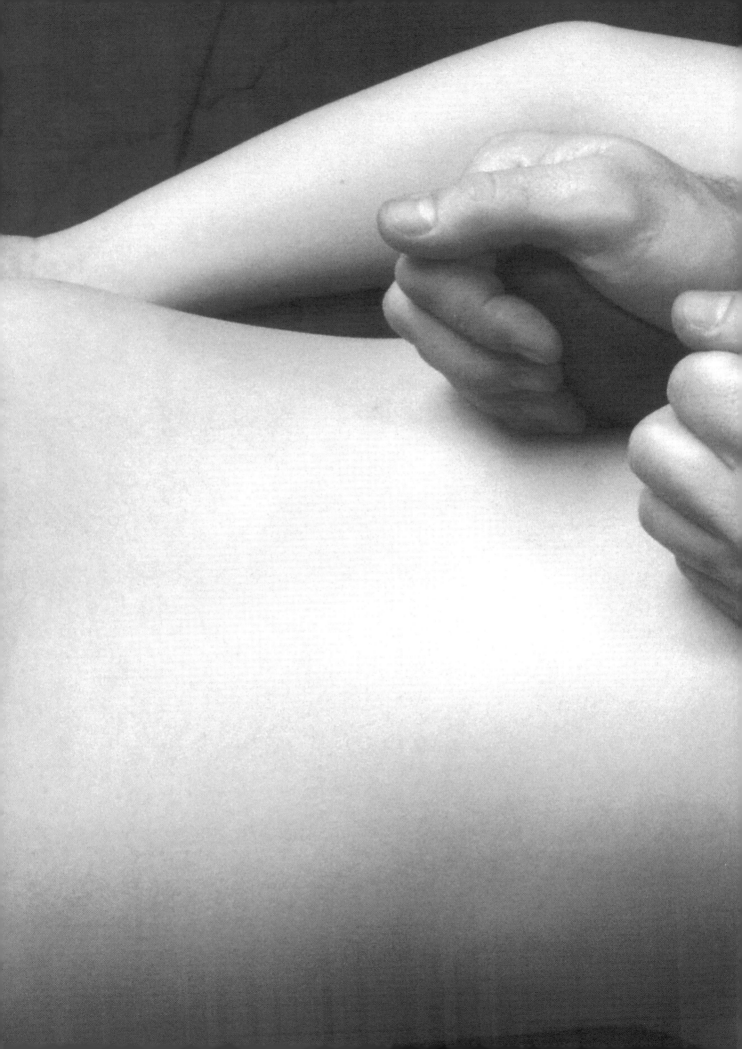

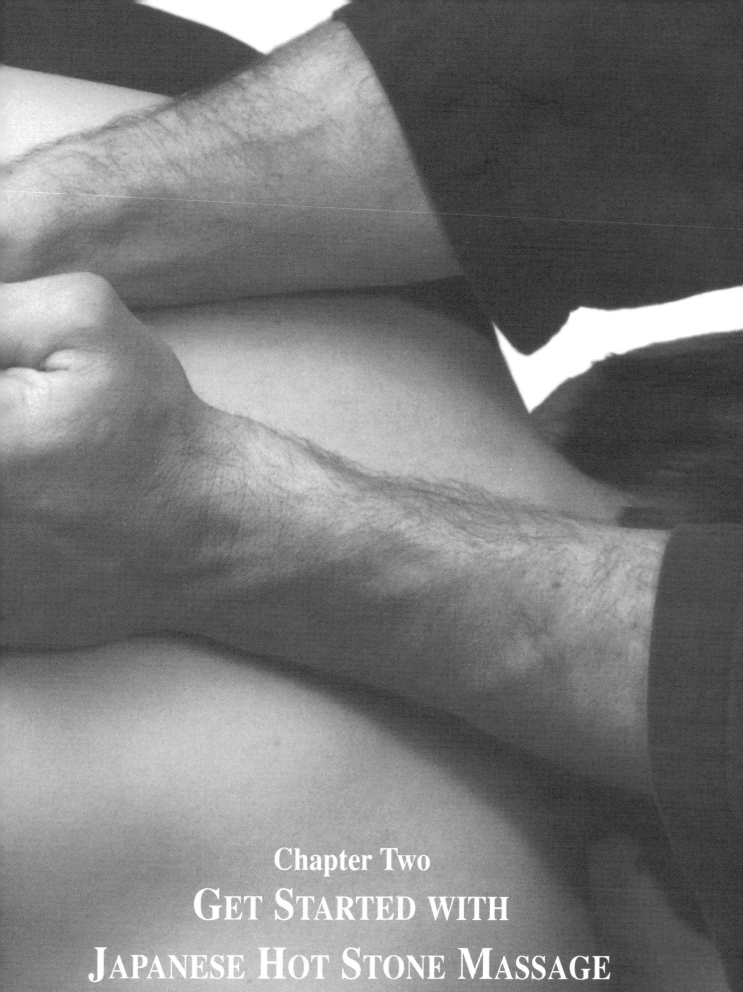

Chapter Two
GET STARTED WITH
JAPANESE HOT STONE MASSAGE

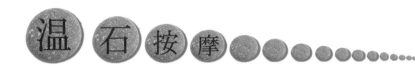

Chapter Two
GET STARTED WITH
JAPANESE HOT STONE MASSAGE

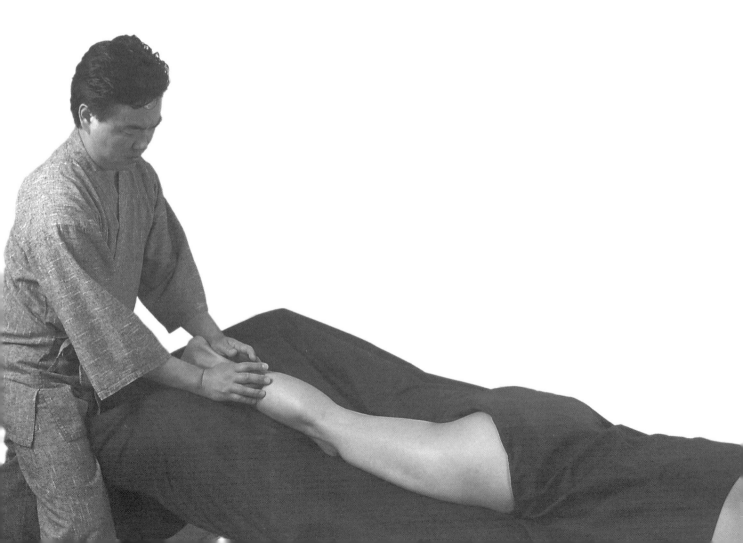

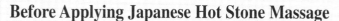

Before Applying Japanese Hot Stone Massage

We recommend that you follow these simple guidelines:

1. To avoid cutting your client and spreading bacterial or fungal infections, keep your fingernails short.
2. Keep your hands and stones clean. Wash your hands with antibacterial soap between each treatment.
3. Remove any jewelry (especially metals) when applying massage, so tendons in your wrists and fingers are not restricted.
4. Warm up, stretch and massage your fingers, hands and arms.
5. Inquire if your client has had any recent injuries, surgery and/or health problems.
6. Inquire if your client has any communicable diseases that you should be aware of, such as flu or tuberculosis.
7. Relax the client and yourself.
8. Your hands should be warm for the initial contact.

Your client should

1. Remove any jewelry.
2. Avoid receiving treatment while extremely hungry or full.

Do not apply massage if your client suffers from

1. A fever
2. A contagious illness
3. Having had recent surgery
4. Skin infections

Other precautions are very similar to those taken in normal professional massage practices. We assume that you understand these professional standards. Have your client consult a doctor if you or the client are in doubt about a medical condition.

After Japanese Hot Stone Massage Treatment

Drinking water after the treatment helps the client eliminate toxins from their body. It is essential that your client drink about two cups of warm water. If your client has heart, liver or kidney disease, this amount should be reduced to about three-quarters of a cup. Tea, coffee, soda or even juices are not good substitutes. Warm water is ideal, though water at room temperature is also acceptable. Cold water chills the internal organs and decreases circulation. If your client does not drink enough water, toxins will stay in the bloodstream and your treatment will be less effective.

After a massage, your client may feel experience some soreness. If this is the case, you are probably working too deep. In the future, moderate the amount of pressure that you apply. If your client requires deep, therapeutic work, they should drink a sufficient amount of water, which will reduce soreness.

Duration and Frequency of Treatment

Just as doctors prescribe medications, it is important to adjust the dosage and frequency of your therapeutic treatments.

Japanese Hot Stone Massage is designed for 50-90 minute treatments. You can also apply shorter 25-30 minute treatments as needed; however, because clients only begin to relax after 15 minutes of treatment, longer treatments are generally more effective. The duration and intensity of your treatment is similar to prescribing a dose of medication. As a professional, you must be able to precisely adjust your treatment to accommodate the age, personal needs and health condition of your client. Massages that last more than 90 minutes drain both the therapist and the client. If you are unable to complete the treatment in one session, schedule another appointment with the client. Generally, 50 to 90 minutes is a comfortable amount of time for a Japanese Hot Stone Massage treatment.

For any medicine or treatment to be effective, the frequency of application is very important. You must adjust the intensity of your treatment according to the frequency of your client's massages. Receiving short treatments once or twice a week is more beneficial than receiving a long massage only once a month. When clients receive frequent massages, they are less likely to accumulate tension; therefore, it takes less time for you to reduce tension and you can apply more therapeutic treatments.

Applying Japanese Hot Stone Massage once or twice each week should keep your client in an optimal, healthy condition. It's okay if someone partakes in several treatments per week, as a luxury. If, however, a client's poor health condition requires such frequent visits, the client should receive other medical treatments or undergo stress management to combat their excess tension.

Special Precautions

Precautions must be taken when applying Japanese Hot Stone Massage on the elderly or people with injuries or illnesses. These precautions are identical to those taken in any other professional massage environment. Due to the heat of the stones, however, special caution must be taken for elderly people and those with very sensitive skin. In these circumstances, it is best to lower the stone temperature and to apply slow, gentle strokes. When working with these types of clients, shorter, more frequent treatments are generally most effective. For instance, two thirty-minute sessions within one given week would be more effective than one fifty-minute treatment.

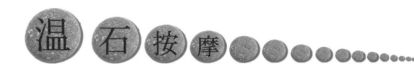

Equipment for Japanese Hot Stone Massage

Japanese Hot Stone Massage requires very few materials if we assume that some bodywork equipment, such as a massage table and sheets, is already in place. In addition, Japanese Hot Stone Massage requires a warming element for the stones. There are several warmers currently available from bodywork supply companies. With a little leg work, however, you can also use a turkey roaster or metal-lined crock pot for the purpose of heating stones. A hot cubby, which is used to heat and steam towels, is also an option.

Like many traditional Japanese massage modalities, Japanese Hot Stone Massage does not typically use lubricants. Japanese massage is traditionally applied over draping or clothing, but when working directly on the skin, powder is used to provide sufficient glide. Powder is advantageous, because you can firmly grip the underlying tissues and manipulate the muscles. We suggest that you use cornstarch, rice powder or powdered honey instead of talc, which can be problematic for some people.

You will also need a set of basalt river stones. Basalt stones are traditionally used in Japan, but they are very expensive to import. Japanese basalt river stones are much darker and smoother than those found in Mexico or the United States. You must use basalt stones, because they retain heat for a longer period of time and will not explode when heated. Stones can be purchased from your local rock quarry or landscaping business. If you live in the appropriate regions and are ambitious, you can also select your stones directly from the source.

Basalt and other volcanic stones can generally withstand the temperatures required for Japanese Hot Stone Massage. However, heating the stones to extreme temperatures (for sanitization or other purposes) when their inner core is still wet could cause a violent explosion. Also avoid heating gem stones, because they are incapable of retaining or withstanding significant temperatures and can easily break or explode.

Size of Stones

Stone size depends on the size of your hands, the size of your client and the technique you are applying. We generally use two sizes of stones—small/medium and medium/large. Small/medium stones are approximately 2–2 1/2" in diameter and should fit into the palm of your hand when it's cupped. The medium/large stones are approximately 3–3 1/2" in diameter and should fit in your open palm, from your thenar eminence to the base of your fingers. Smaller stones don't retain heat as long, but they can fit into specific muscle locations. Larger stones retain the heat more efficiently and can cover significant areas, so they are used on large muscle groups.

How to Sanitize Your Stones

Follow the same procedures to sanitize new stones and those you have used during previous treatments. Place the stones in a sink with warm water and one ounce of bio-degradable liquid soap or dish detergent. Scrub each individual stone with a brillo pad, then rinse them thoroughly and place them on a clean towel. Next, spray each stone with a 50% water/50% rubbing alcohol solution and wipe them clean.

After each cleaning, allow the stones to dry overnight. Stones are natural, which means that each surface will have some irregularities. Thorough air drying will complete the sanitization process, by allowing moisture to evaporate from the porous surface of the stones. Store the stones in salt, used for purification in Japan, which will keep them clean and dry for longer periods of time.

For daily Japanese Hot Stone Massage treatments, fill your stone warming apparatus with enough water to cover the stones and add 1/4 teaspoon of Spa Oxidizer. You can purchase Spa Oxidizer from any pool and hot tub supply business or large hardware store. Spa Oxidizer will sufficiently sanitize the stones for a day full of treatments.

Special circumstances may require more extensive stone sanitization. If the client's skin is questionable, spray the stones with alcohol and wipe each stone before returning it to the warmer. You may also sprinkle salt directly into the stone warmer during treatments. In the worst case, change the water at the end of the treatment and add more Spa Oxidizer. At the end of each day clean out the stone warmer and sanitize the stones by following the above procedures.

How to Heat Your Stones

Stone temperature should remain at 130°F, regardless of the dial control readings on your heating element. Use a liquid cooking thermometer, which can be purchased at most grocery or department stores, to maintain the correct temperature. Heat the stones in 130°F water for approximately twenty minutes prior to use. Thoroughly heating the stones before each treatment encourages longer heat retention.

Adjusting Stone Temperature

At the start of the treatment, ensure the stone temperature is correct before contacting the client's body. This temperature is primarily determined by the heat of the stones in your hands. You must remember that our hands are very desensitized, and consider this before applying stones to sensitive areas of your client's skin. It will take moderate practice to precisely adjust the temperature of the stones.

Fresh stones (in this book, "fresh stones" refers to stones that have just been removed from the warmer, not brand new stones) must always be applied with a moving stroke until they are properly acclimated. Fresh stones are much too hot to stay in one place on the client's body for a

Stones can be purchased from Kotobuki Publications: 1-800-651-2662 or **www.japanesemassage.com**

prolonged period of time. When the stone temperature drops and the client's surface tissue and muscles have sufficiently absorbed heat from the stones, you may continue with rotation and vibration techniques.

During the initial strokes and throughout the entire Japanese Hot Stone Massage, you may turn the stones in your hands to maintain an even temperature on both sides. When one side of the stone has cooled, it doesn't necessarily mean that the other side is also cool. The client's tissue will absorb more heat than your hands, which means the stone temperature will be higher on your hands than it is on the client's skin. Less heat may be necessary when using stationary pressure or working on a client with sensitive skin, but never apply these techniques with cold stones. Switch to fresh stones at regular intervals to ensure that your treatment is as comfortable and therapeutic as possible. To maintain fluidity and avoid disruptions during the treatment, you should switch stones while in a transition from one part of the body to the next. If you must switch stones during a technique, avoid interrupting the flow and apply a stroking technique until the stone temperature is appropriate.

Exchanging and Circulating Stones

When exchanging and circulating stones, place them back in the warmer from left to right, so you know which are hottest. Generally, four to six stones are removed at one time. This will limit how often your hands enter the water, and will also minimize the number of times your hands leave the client's body. Since only two stones can be used at one time, keep the other stones in a terry cloth apron or wrapped in towels near the massage table. When the last stones have cooled, return them to the warmer and extract another set.

Dealing with Damp Skin

Applying Japanese Hot Stone Massage on clients with very damp or sweaty skin conditions can be extremely problematic. If the client's skin is slightly damp, you may add a small amount of powder to continue applying the massage. If someone is extremely sweaty or wet, remove the moisture with a towel before applying any powder. If the dampness is a continual problem, apply the entire treatment over draping with slightly warmer stones.

How to Adjust the Amount of Pressure

As with other massage modalities, the amount of pressure used during a massage should be precisely adjusted to each client's condition and sensitivity. If you haven't gained control with the stones, you may have difficulty regulating the pressure, applying it too light or too deep. Japanese Hot Stone Massage can easily be applied using too much pressure, so practice pressure techniques until you can precisely adjust the pressure for each client. Also be careful when moving the stones over bony surfaces, because too much pressure on these areas can be uncomfortable for the client.

How to Practice Japanese Hot Stone Massage

Practice each technique until you feel completely comfortable applying it without analyzing your performance. The goal is to deliver a smooth, comfortable massage without breaking the flow of the treatment. While performing a technique, think about the next technique you will employ, based upon the client's needs and the goals of the session. You cannot interrupt the massage between techniques to think about what you are going to do next. Once you master each example, combine different techniques with smooth transitions to create a seamless hot stone massage.

You don't need to include all fifty-five Japanese Hot Stone Massage techniques within one massage session. You should choose those techniques that work best within each situation. Although you may freely choose the order in which you apply the techniques, there are general guidelines to applying certain Japanese massage techniques. Stroking techniques are often applied to warm the tissues and prepare for deeper work. The majority of the treatment is then done with rotation techniques. Pressure techniques should always be applied toward the end of the massage when the tissues are well-warmed. To safely apply stretching techniques, the tissue must be thoroughly warmed by previous massage techniques. These are traditional guidelines, but you should still work freely and creatively. If you do not follow these guidelines, you will still be able to give a safe, effective massage with these techniques.

Using Lubrication

Japanese Hot Stone Massage techniques are typically applied without lubrication; however, you can apply most of these techniques with oil or other lubricants. Lubricants help the stones retain the heat for a longer period of time; however, it is more difficult to engage the underlying tissue with lubricated stones, which is essential for many of these techniques. When applying significant pressure with lubrication, you must prevent the stones from slipping, which can cause therapist and client injury. Use as little lubrication as possible during your treatment. Regardless of whether you use lubricants, Japanese Hot Stone Massage techniques are very therapeutic and compatible with other therapies.

Incorporating Other Hot Stone Therapies

You don't have to use Japanese Hot Stone Massage techniques exclusively; instead, use a few techniques from this book to enhance your existing hot stone massage treatments. If you currently perform hot stone treatments with oil or other lubricants, be sure the techniques you choose from this book work with lubrication and fit smoothly into your existing treatment.

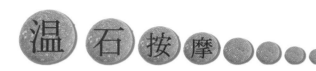

How to Position Your Body

Apply Japanese Hot Stone Massage on a massage table set at a regular height, with your client in either the prone or supine position. It can also be applied in other positions, such as side or sitting positions, but these positions are used for special circumstances, such as pregnancy, when the client is unable to lay on their stomach. Regardless of the setting, place bolsters or cushions beneath the client's knees for added comfort. Professionals who practice an Asian modality and are used to working on the floor may also apply these techniques in that position.

Some techniques are best applied from a standing position, while others should be applied while seated or kneeling to reduce wrist angle and prevent hyperextension. Your height and the height of the massage table will determine the best working position. Find the most safe and comfortable position from which to apply these techniques. Proper body position is explained in Step 1 of each technique, but feel free to modify these positions as necessary.

A peaceful and quiet environment can also enhance the massage. It is best to apply the massage in a warm, quiet room. Interruptions and noises, such as phone calls, should be reduced or eliminated. Soft, soothing music can also facilitate relaxation. If you are in a cooler environment, have a sheet or blanket available to keep your client warm. When clients turn to the supine position, they often feel chilled. It is very important that the room is warm and your client is properly covered to avoid any discomfort.

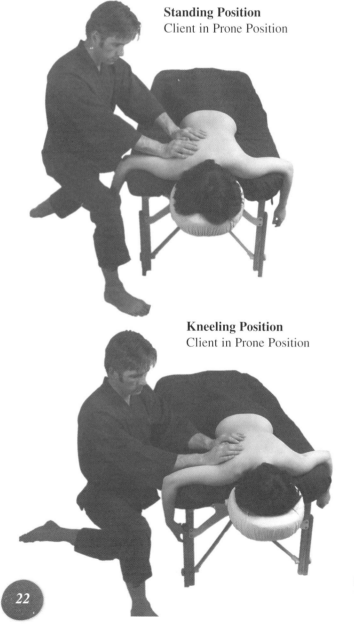

Standing Position
Client in Prone Position

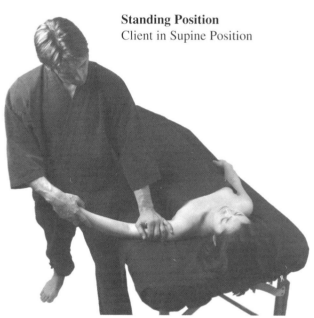

Standing Position
Client in Supine Position

Kneeling Position
Client in Prone Position

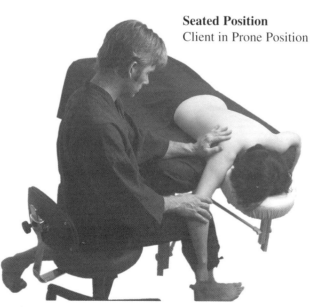

Seated Position
Client in Prone Position

Proper Body Mechanics

Proper body mechanics improve your overall massage therapy practice, therefore increasing your income. Proper body mechanics reduce tension and stress, allowing you to perform higher quality massages. If you are not physically or mentally prepared for a massage, clients will sense your hesitation and lack of energy. Improper body mechanics make your treatments less effective, which ultimately damages your massage career, by reducing your return and regular clients.

Seven Rules For Improving Body Mechanics:
These seven tips will improve the quality of your massage, by minimizing stress to your body.

1. Lower and widen your body stance.
Keep your legs wide and your feet perpendicular. This stable stance evenly distributes your body weight and facilitates fluid movement. A wide stance prevents leaning during long strokes. If you are unable to apply long strokes without leaning over, separate the stroke into two sections to ensure smoothness and create less stress on your body.

2. Open your chest and shoulders to improve *ki* flow.
Leaning forward causes your chest and shoulders to curve inward, which creates stress in your back and shoulders. When you hunch over, *ki* can not move from the *hara* (abdomen) through the chest and out to the arms. This posture also restricts air *ki* intake and lung movement, which reduces your overall *ki* energy.

3. Relax your shoulders, elbows, wrists and entire body.
When you are relaxed, your movements are smooth and fluid; however, tension makes your treatment rigid and uncomfortable. Experienced therapists can deliver fluid massages from the subconscious brain, which is smoother, requires less effort and is more enjoyable for clients. Regardless of how new you are to the profession, you must remember to relax.

4. Pull rather than push.
"Whenever you can push, you can always pull" is a traditional Asian bodywork concept, which is different from Western techniques. Applying techniques from the opposite direction or from across the body, will prevent joint compression. Compressing while pushing creates grinding stress on your cartilage and leads to permanent wrist, elbow or shoulder pain. Thousands of dollars spent on massage education and building your practice, along with time and effort put into becoming a therapist, are all at risk due to improper body mechanics.

5. Your massage should be an even exercise.
Many massage therapists exercise only their arms, hands and upper body during treatments. Correct posture disperses your movements through several muscle groups, instead of overworking one individual area. At the end of a massage, you will feel more balanced and energized, instead of aching and tired. This concept is especially important when you perform four or five massages per day.

6. Own the right equipment and set it up correctly.
A good, solid, yet comfortable, massage table is worth every single penny that you pay for it. Less expensive, imported equipment often squeaks, wobbles and is unsafe and uncomfortable for your clients. A solid table will ultimately improve the quality of your massage practice.

Adjusting your table to the correct height will drastically impact and improve your overall health. A table set too high is stressful for your neck and shoulders, while a table set too low is stressful for your lower back. Use the massage table to balance and stabilize your body weight. Wedge your knees beneath the table or rest your pelvis against the table for support.

Heat therapy equipment helps soften muscles before you work on them. Towel warmers or heating pads are very good investments and will help reduce muscle tension. This also reduces time spent on tight muscles and softens hard surfaces, like the bottom of the feet.

7. Daily maintenance for your body.
You should always practice hand, wrist and arm maintenance. Daily self-massage is especially important before your first client in order to properly warm your hands and arms. If your muscles and tendons are inflexible during a massage, one wrong move can cause hand or wrist injury.

To improve your body mechanics, you must partake in daily activities, such as exercise, yoga or tai chi, to keep yourself in optimal shape. Receiving massages also makes you aware of your own body tension and maintains optimal condition.

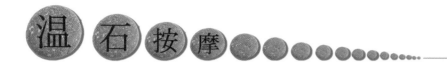

Techniques to Avoid

Many professional massage therapists complain of problems in their hands or fingers. Japanese Hot Stone Massage is beneficial, because it creates less stress for your hands and fingers than other Western massage modalities. Western styles of massage and reflexology often contain movements that are extremely stressful for the hands and fingers. Any pain or discomfort generally indicates excessive wrist or elbow stress. You must pay careful attention to these warning signs. Never work through the pain; it will lead to permanent joint problems and will jeopardize your career. Readjust to find the most correct, comfortable position. Protecting yourself is always the first priority. The following are some common mistakes made when applying Japanese Hot Stone Massage and how to correct them.

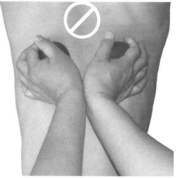

1) Do not hyperadduct your wrists. Hyperadduction creates compression between the ulna and carpal bones. This will eventually lead to painful nerve compression. This position is also very stressful for the pectoralis muscles.

Hyperadducting the wrists

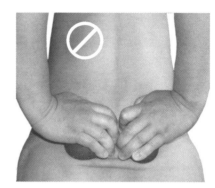

3) Do not hyperabduct your wrists. Hyperabduction creates compression between radius and carpal bones. This will eventually lead to painful nerve compression and other problems.

Hyperabducting the wrists

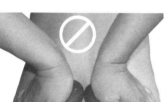

2) Do not hyperextend your wrists, even momentarily. Hyperextending your wrists can create severe problems in the muscles, ligaments, tendons and fascia in the wrist. You must maintain a safe wrist angle at all times.

Hyperextending the wrists

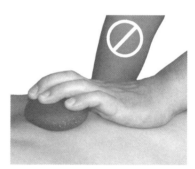

4) Do not hyperextend the metacarpophalangeal joints. Applying heavy downward pressure while holding the stones under your fingers can hyperextend the metacarpophalangeal joints.

Hyperextending the metacarpophalangeal joints

Finding the Best Position

This entire book is written for the average-sized therapist working on the average-sized client in healthy condition. If you are not comfortable with a particular technique, or if a technique makes your client uncomfortable, slightly adjust your body angle or reduce the amount of pressure. Check your body position to ensure that you are relaxed during application. You or your client may still be uncomfortable with a technique, even after you have approached it in a variety of ways. If this is the case, it is best to omit the technique altogether. If applying a technique creates any hand or wrist stress, slightly change the angle of your hand to find an easier position. Remember, each therapist's body is slightly different and adjustments may be necessary. Even if you omit several techniques from your repertoire, you will have enough remaining to give a superlative massage. No technique is ever worth risking injury to your hands or body.

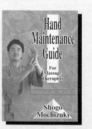

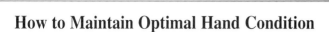

How to Maintain Optimal Hand Condition

Many hand problems can be prevented, reduced or eliminated by performing a daily maintenance massage on your own hands and forearms. Massage is a physical exercise; just as you stretch and warm up before any other physical activities, you must massage and stretch your hands before giving a massage. When working for several hours at a time, you must frequently massage and stretch your hands. This is especially important when you feel tightness in your hands and forearms, which often occurs the morning after a day of giving multiple massages. You must properly warm and loosen your muscles before performing a massage. Spend about five minutes massaging and stretching your fingers, hands, wrists, arms and shoulders before and after each massage. This will prevent the majority of injuries that occur from repetitive improper movements or from forcing inflexible muscles and tendons. We teach our students a complete hand maintenance routine; here are a few examples of the most important techniques.

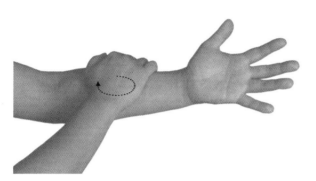

1. Palm Rotation on the Forearm

Place your left arm on the massage table with your palm facing up. Place the heel of your right hand over the forearm flexors, just distal to your elbow. Apply pressure with the heel of your hand to engage the underlying tissue. Apply small rotations for three to five seconds. Slightly reposition your hand distally and repeat until you cover the entire anterior surface of your forearm. Reverse hands and apply the technique to your right arm.

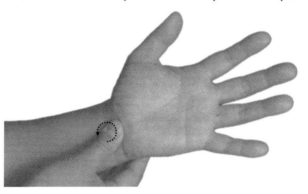

3. Thumb Rotation on the Wrist

Place your thumb on the inner side of the wrist, just below the other thumb, and wrap your fingers behind the wrist for support. Apply rotation by using your entire hand (not just the thumb). Move the thumb across the middle of your wrist, working your way to the hypothenar side of your hand and repeat the rotation. Repeat on the other wrist as well.

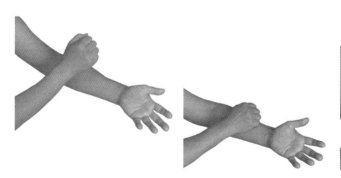

2. Percussion on the Forearm

Make a soft, loose fist with your right hand. Apply percussion to your forearm with the loose fist, keeping your wrist very loose as well. You can strike with the front of your fist (as pictured), the side of your wrist or the back of your hand. Apply percussion over a particular area for a sustained period of time, then slightly reposition distally and repeat. Continue repositioning and repeat the technique until you have covered your entire forearm. Reverse hands and apply the technique to your right arm.

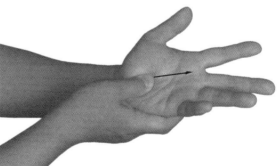

4. Stroking Between the Metacarpals

Place your thumb on the heel of your hand and wrap your fingers behind the hand for support. Slowly stroke your thumb between the metacarpal bones. Begin just above the wrist and end between the base of each finger. Work between all of the metacarpals, including the space between the thumb and index finger. Repeat on the dorsal side. Use lubrication if needed.

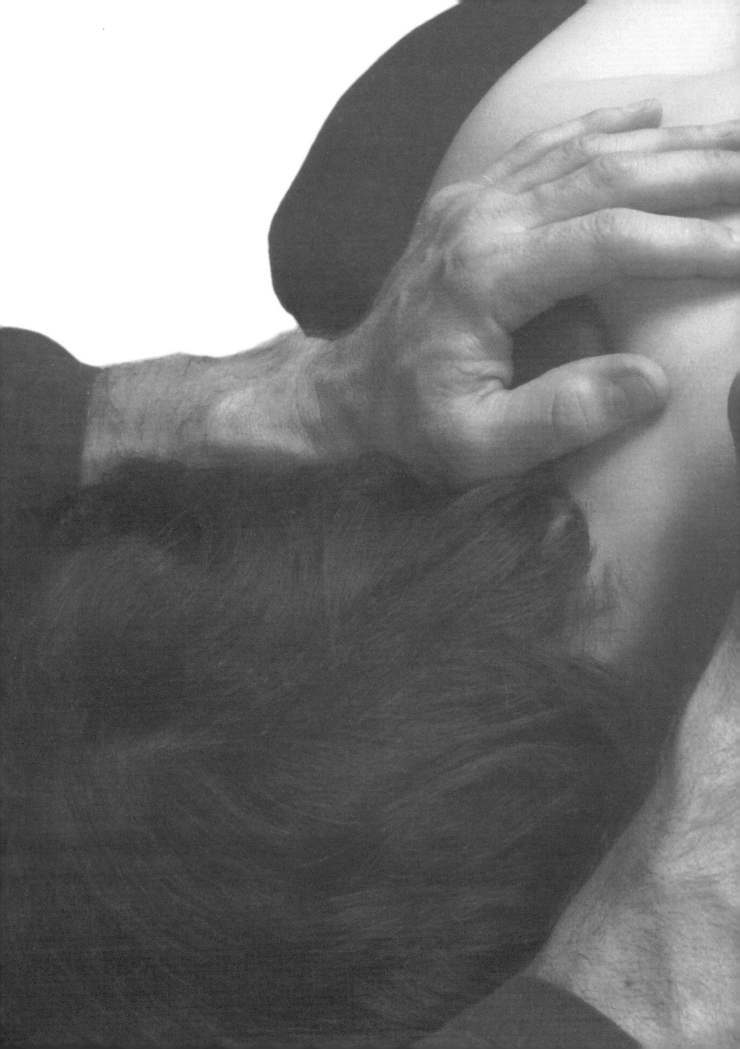

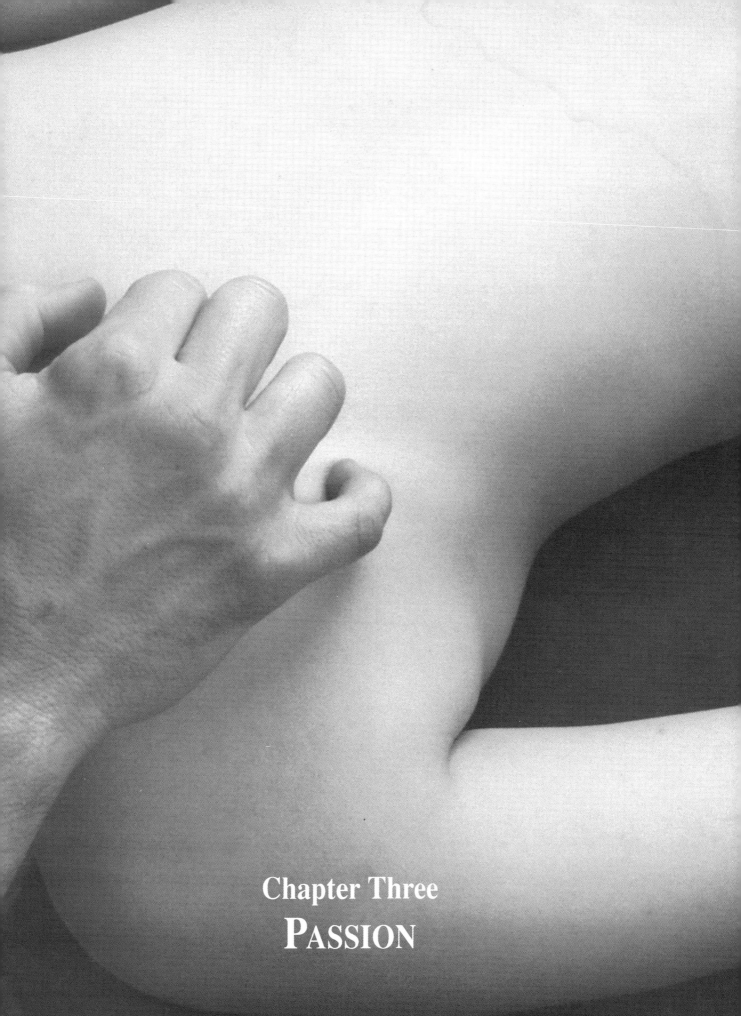

Chapter Three
PASSION

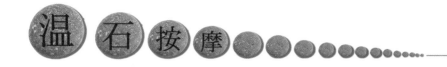

Chapter Three
PASSION
Techniques for the Posterior Upper Extremities

In this chapter, we introduce twenty Japanese Hot Stone Massage techniques for the back, neck and shoulders. The first stage of treatment introduces the fire element, which represents emotions and actions of passion. Passion is the most important part of treating the human body. In popular society, passion is most often expressed in upper body actions. These techniques are applied while the client is lying on the massage table in the prone position, using the face cradle. Place a bolster beneath the ankles and cover your client with sheets from the waist down. Ensure that your client is completely comfortable.

The first five techniques are used to warm the body. These techniques are broken down individually by description; however, they should be incorporated into your own massage sequence. The beginning and end of a massage are the most important aspects. Your first touch will set the tone for the entire treatment. If your client gets a negative first impression, their body and mind resist treatment, and your entire massage will be less effective. Your first touch should be smooth, and the stone temperature should be comfortable and soothing for your client.

The second set of five techniques focuses on the upper shoulder region. Upper shoulder tension is one of the most common problems faced in modern living. Your ability to effectively reduce and manage your client's upper back tension will ensure return clients and maintain the success of your practice.

The third set of four examples introduces techniques for the upper arms, shoulders and sides of the torso. People who are

athletes, or those who have physically demanding occupations, tend to have extremely tight shoulder and rotator cuff muscles. If these muscles are not very tight, the duration of these specific techniques may be limited accordingly.

The last set of six techniques addresses the low back and upper gluteal region. Over seventy percent of Americans have or have had low back problems during their lives. If your client has a herniated or bulging disc, some of these techniques should be avoided. If the lower back is simply tight, these techniques will help reduce tension and encourage a healthy low back condition. To effectively treat the low back, you must also address hip, leg and mid-back tension. Due to the reciprocal and compensatory relationship between muscles in this region, muscle tension will not release until all primary tensions are addressed. After you understand Japanese Hot Stone Massage, you may seamlessly combine low back techniques with those for the legs and hips to more effectively address low back conditions.

A fresh set of hot stones should be introduced at the beginning of each section, or as the stones cool. Use the stroking techniques at the beginning of each section to properly adjust the temperature of the stones. If the stones cool too quickly, you must introduce new stones in the middle of the section. Remember to apply the stroking techniques again until the stones are at an adequate temperature. You do not have to apply these techniques in the order in which they are presented; however, this sequence will help until you develop your own routine.

温石按摩

Meridians in the Posterior Trunk

Please note that when an internal organ is capitalized, it refers to the Asian form of the organ. Asian and Western ideas of internal organ function are often quite different. This book briefly introduces meridians, but for further information about meridians, tsubo and their functions, please refer to *Shiatsu for the Hand* and *Shiatsu for the Foot*.

Large Intestine Meridian

The Large Intestine Meridian's main function is elimination of food waste. In Asian medicine, the Large Intestine also helps the Lungs, which take in heaven essence.

San Sho (Triple Heater) Meridian

San sho does not have a material equivalent in Western physiology, but it is an important meridian, and helps balance and regulate the temperature within the trunk of the body. *San sho* is also important for protecting and supporting Heart function.

Small Intestine Meridian

The Small Intestine Meridian's main function is taking nutrients and earth essence from the food. The Heart is the combustion chamber for *ki* energy and the Small Intestine Meridian supports the creation of primary functioning *ki* energy.

Bladder Meridian

The Bladder's main function is collecting and eliminating liquid waste. The Bladder channel is also responsible for balancing all meridians. For instance, when a person is moderately off balance, this often indicates an problem with the Bladder Meridian. The Kidney and Bladder are both water elements and the Bladder supports Kidney function.

Governing Vessel

The Governing Vessel runs along the median line on the posterior trunk, beginning at the anus, following directly along the spine, over the top of the nose and ending in the mouth. The primary function of the Governing Vessel is to maintain an energetic balance in all *yang* meridians.

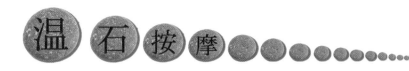

温石軽擦法
Light Stroking Over the Entire Back

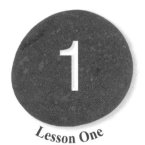

Lesson One

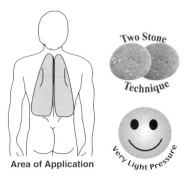

Area of Application

Two Stone Technique

Very Light Pressure

Begin Japanese Hot Stone Massage with smooth, gentle strokes over the entire back. Warming the tissue is an essential preparation for deep massage applications. It is important to ensure that the stone temperature is comfortable and tolerable for your client. The beginning of a massage is most important, because it sets the tone for the entire procedure. Apply a small amount of powder to the client's skin to smoothly apply this stroke. Repeat this technique until the stones are cool enough for slower stroking techniques. Correct body mechanics and posture are essential for giving an effective massage. Proper posture not only helps avoid injury and stress to your body, it improves the overall quality of your massage.

Stand at the end of the table by the face cradle. We recommend that you use a stance, in which your feet are placed in a large perpendicular pattern. This position distributes your body weight and lowers your hips to reduce wrist angle during application. Your individual body position will depend on your height and the length of your arms. Avoid contacting the face cradle with any part of your body (besides your hands) to prevent client discomfort.

St1ep

- Stand by the face cradle in a stable stance.
- Place your palms with stones over the rhomboid minor muscles.
- Relax your wrists and fingers, while keeping them relatively straight.
- Hold the stones in your palms, so there is no extra stress on your wrists.

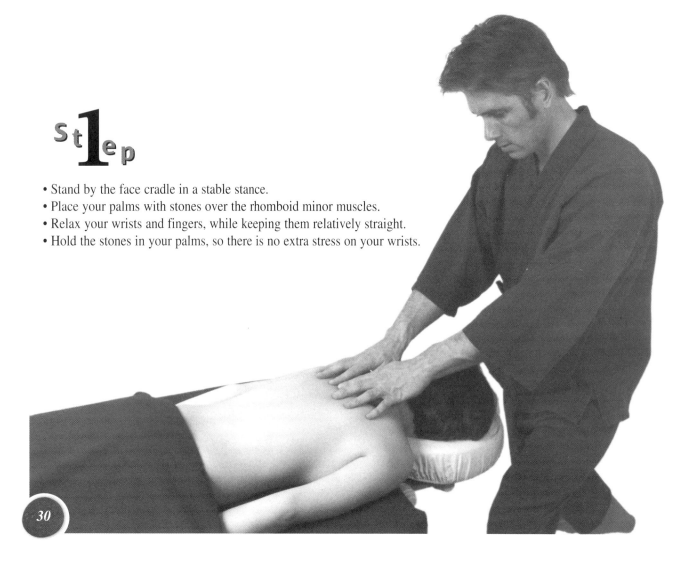

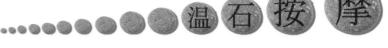

- Stroke inferiorly over the erector muscles toward the hips.
- Stroke parallel to the spine, but do not contact the spine or scapula.
- Stroke using your body movement, not hand and wrist strength.

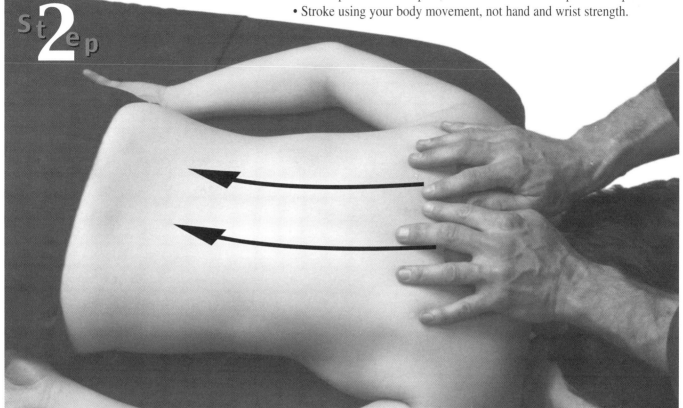

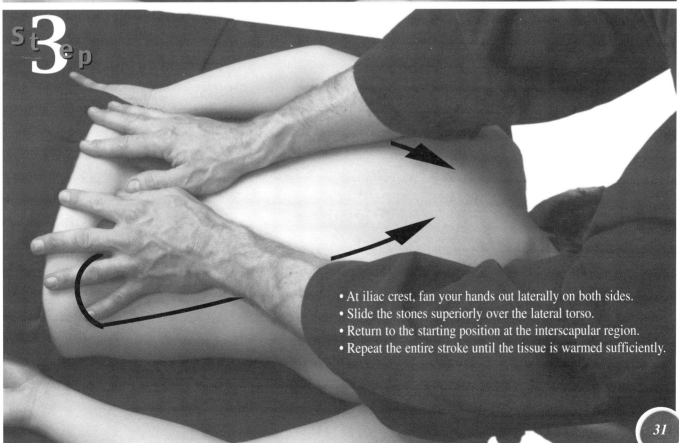

- At iliac crest, fan your hands out laterally on both sides.
- Slide the stones superiorly over the lateral torso.
- Return to the starting position at the interscapular region.
- Repeat the entire stroke until the tissue is warmed sufficiently.

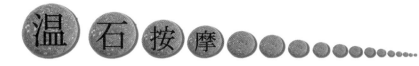

温石軽擦法
Deep Stroking Over the Lamina Groove

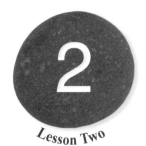

Lesson Two

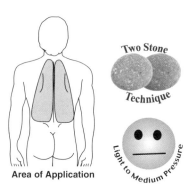

Area of Application

Two Stone Technique

Light to Medium Pressure

After warming the back with the previous technique, apply slow, relatively deep strokes over the lamina groove and entire thoracic. Move the stones much slower during this technique, allowing the heat to penetrate more efficiently. The stones must be acclimated by the previous technique to avoid client discomfort. Use proper body mechanics to reduce the risk of elbow or wrist injuries. As you perform this technique, do not lean forward or rely solely upon upper body strength. Instead, lower your stance and move your entire body forward to support this movement. If your shoulders or forearms feel stress during application, this generally indicates that your posture is incorrect. To maintain proper body mechanics, bend your knees and slightly lower your stance. If the stones don't slide smoothly, your body position may be too high or your client's skin may be too damp. Either lower your stance or apply more powder.

Step 1

- Stand by the face cradle in a stable stance.
- Place your palms with stones over the rhomboid minor muscles.
- Drop your elbows to minimize wrist stress.

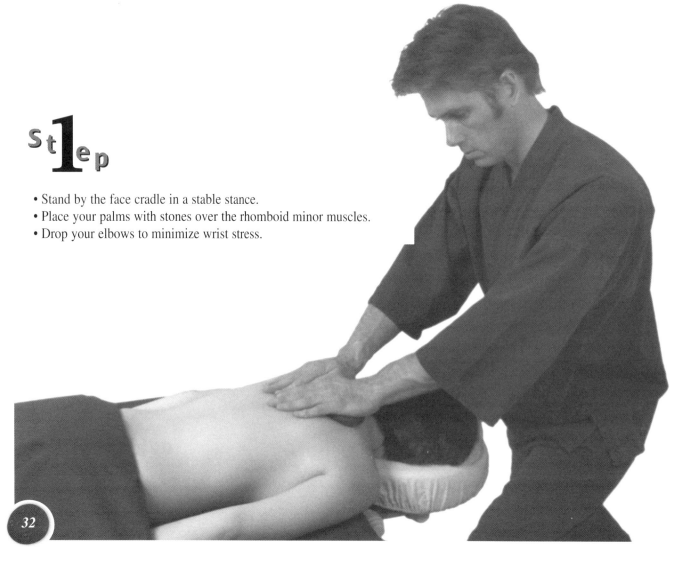

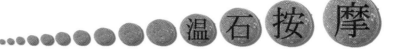

Step 2

- Stroke inferiorly over the lamina groove toward the hips.
- Stroke relatively slow with sufficient pressure.
- Stroke parallel to the spine, but do not contact the spine or scapula with the stones.
- Hook the edges of the stones into the heels of your palms for smooth application.

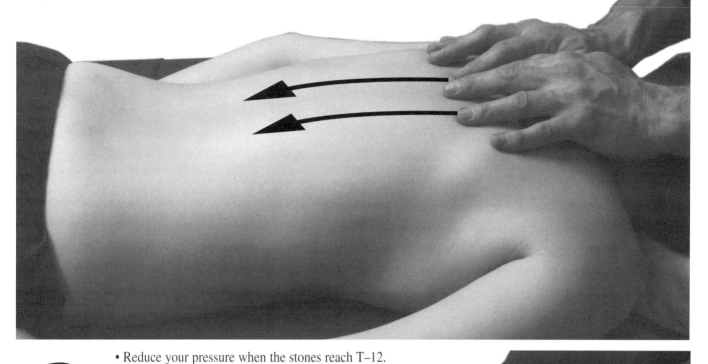

Step 3

- Reduce your pressure when the stones reach T–12.
- When you reach the iliac crest, fan the stones out laterally.
- Stroke the stones superiorly over the lateral torso.
- Return to the starting position in the interscapular region.
- Repeat two to three times, or as necessary.

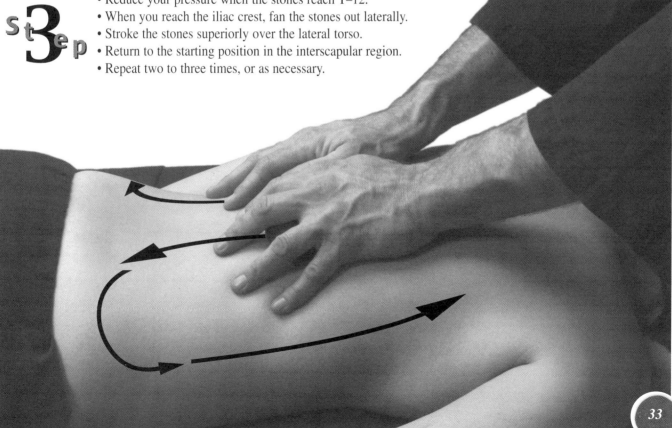

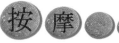

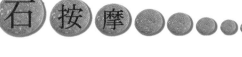 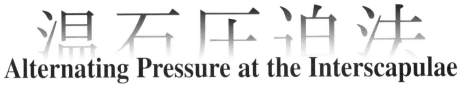

③

Lesson Three

Alternating Pressure at the Interscapulae

Area of Application

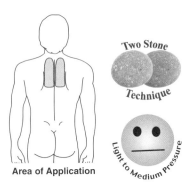

Two Stone Technique

Light to Medium Pressure

The interscapular region of the upper shoulders is one of the most common places to carry tension. After loosening the client's entire back, you can begin reducing tension within the interscapular region. The rhomboid muscles, along with the erector muscles in the neck, experience a significant amount of tension. Apply this pressure technique on both sides of the spine, using alternating pressure to initially reduce muscle tension. In Asian bodywork, muscle tension is released from the center of the body out to the tips of the limbs, which is opposite the typical Western method for releasing muscle tension. Before you can effectively loosen neck or rotator cuff muscles, you must loosen the interscapular region. To ensure that you do not use excessive pressure during this technique, adjust the pressure according to your client's sensitivity. You should never feel stress in your wrists, and if your wrists or shoulders are experiencing tension, you must readjust your body mechanics.

Step 1

- Stand by the face cradle in a stable stance.
- Place your lower palms with stones over the rhomboid minor muscles.
- Drop your elbows to reduce wrist stress.

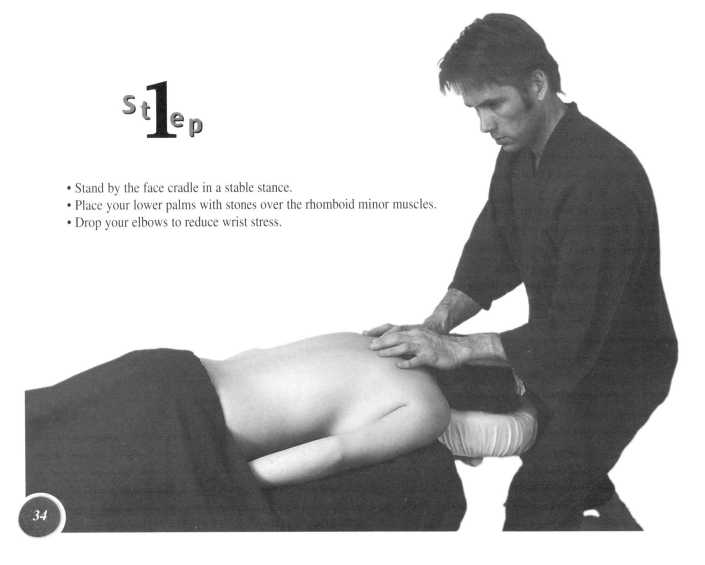

温石按摩

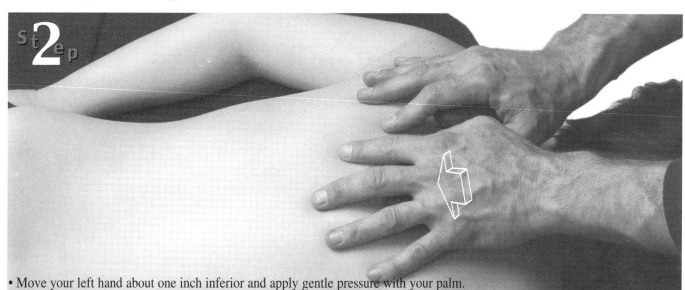

• Move your left hand about one inch inferior and apply gentle pressure with your palm.

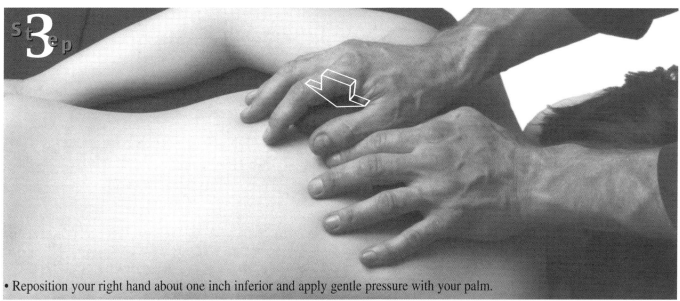

• Reposition your right hand about one inch inferior and apply gentle pressure with your palm.

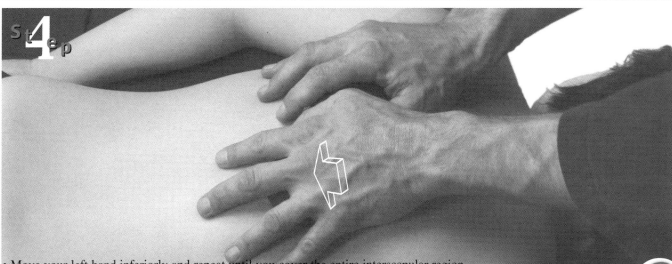

• Move your left hand inferiorly and repeat until you cover the entire interscapular region.
• Repeat the entire procedure as necessary.

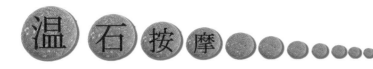

Japanese Hot Stone Massage

Light Pressure on the Interscapular Region

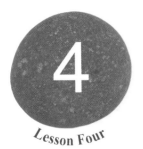

Lesson Four

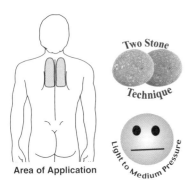

Area of Application

Two Stone Technique

Light to Medium Pressure

We will now address the interscapular region with this deep pressure technique, which involves hooking and pulling superiorly into the underlying tissue. Before applying this technique, be sure the interscapular region has been properly warmed by the previous techniques, especially Lesson #3. Western massage, which is typically stroke-based, focuses less on understanding muscle characteristics than East Asian therapy.

Asian bodywork is typically a kneading or pressure-based massage, which involves engaging the underlying tissue and requires very specific manipulations. Therefore, when performing Asian bodywork, it is important to understand each muscle's characteristics. For instance, when stretching or applying pressure to the rhomboid muscles, we separate the muscle by pulling upwards. Adjust the amount of pressure and never apply techniques that are uncomfortable for the client. If, however, if you don't use enough pressure, the treatment will lack therapeutic value. With experience, you can more accurately determine the appropriate amount of pressure according to the technique and your client. Regardless of your skill level and experience, you must maintain open communication with your client.

Step 1

- Kneel or sit in a chair next to the face cradle.
- Hold the stones with the edges protruding from the hypothenar side.
- Place your hands with stones at the inferior edge of the rhomboid major.

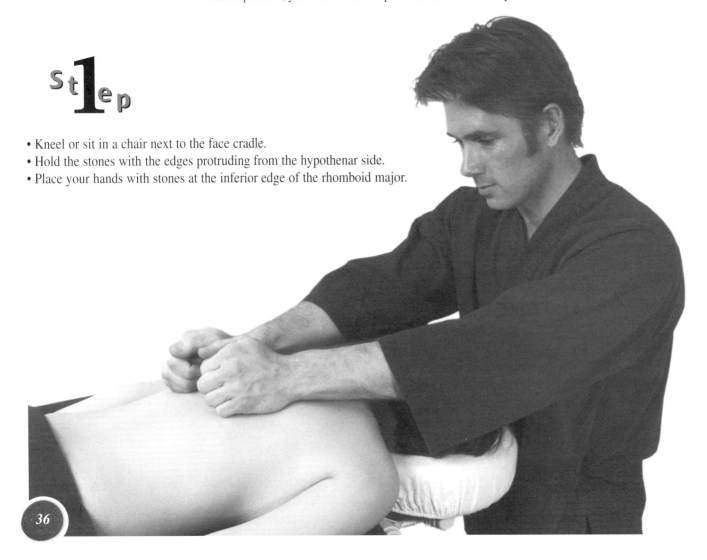

36

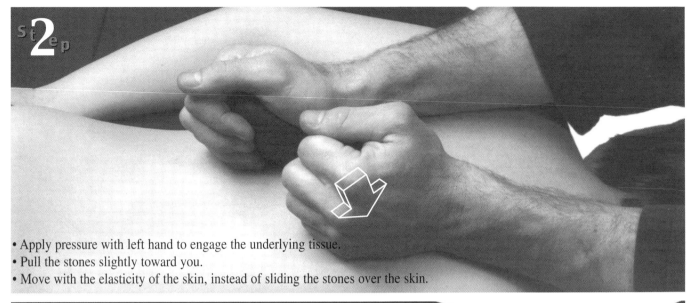

- Apply pressure with left hand to engage the underlying tissue.
- Pull the stones slightly toward you.
- Move with the elasticity of the skin, instead of sliding the stones over the skin.

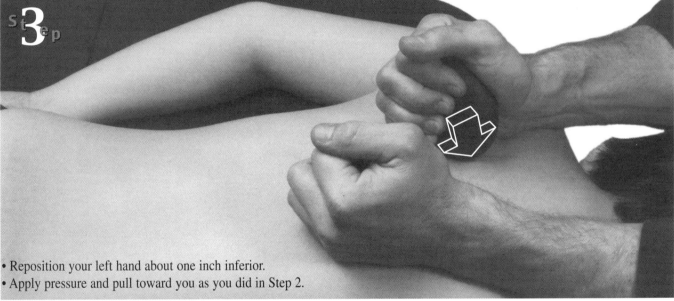

- Reposition your left hand about one inch inferior.
- Apply pressure and pull toward you as you did in Step 2.

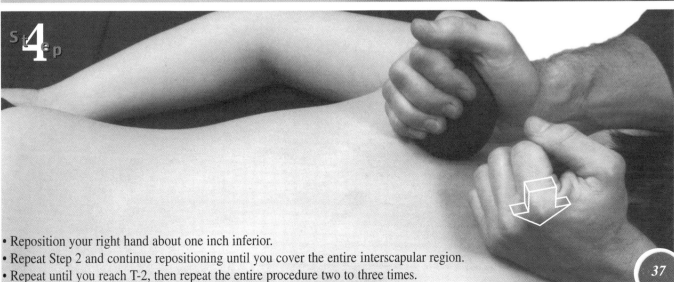

- Reposition your right hand about one inch inferior.
- Repeat Step 2 and continue repositioning until you cover the entire interscapular region.
- Repeat until you reach T-2, then repeat the entire procedure two to three times.

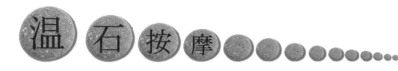

Lesson Five

温石軽擦法
Circular Stroking Over the Scapula

This light stroking technique is an introduction and transition that acclimates the tissue for the next series of techniques. When applying Lessons #5-11, lightly stroke to adjust the stone temperature, acclimate the underlying tissue and maintain therapeutic levels of heat. Each time you introduce fresh hot stones, use this technique until they cool to an appropriate temperature, before applying deeper, more focused and localized techniques. The speed of this stroke is determined by the temperature of your stones: warmer stones must move quickly and continually until they are acclimated, before proceeding to the next technique. Apply light strokes periodically throughout the massage to maintain an overall layer of heat on the body. Alternate between the left and right trapezius to release tension evenly and allow the tissue to rest and recuperate between strokes. Alternating your strokes in this fashion also assists in moving toxins into the blood and other fluids for elimination.

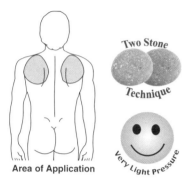

Area of Application

Two Stone
Technique

Very Light Pressure

Step 1

- Kneel or sit in a chair next to the face cradle.
- Place both palms with stones on the superior interscapular region.
- Stroke the entire back in the same manner as Lesson #1.
- Reach as far as possible without overextending yourself.
- Drop and relax your elbows and shoulders.
- You may also stand while applying this technique.

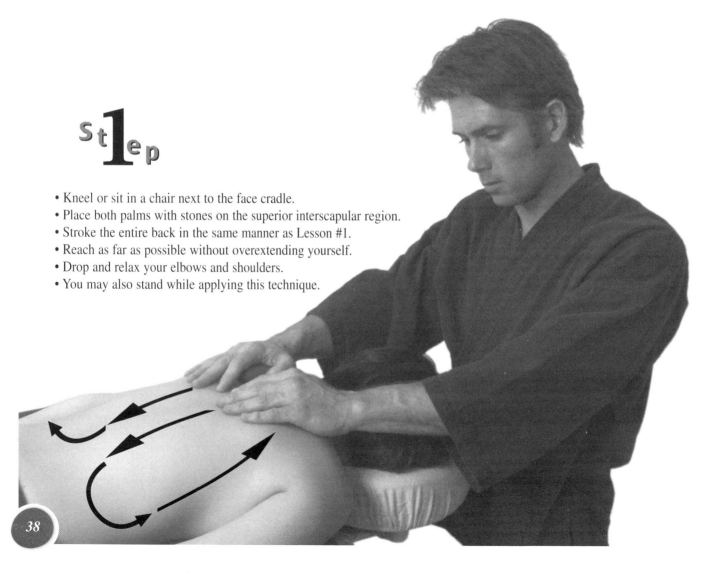

st**2**ep
• Continue light, smooth strokes over the shoulder blades, without creating client discomfort.
• Move inferiorly over the interscapular region, then laterally toward the axillary region to create a circular motion.

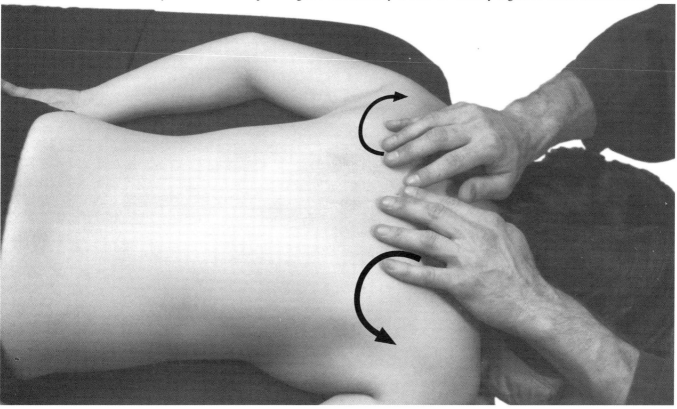

st**3**ep
• Continue the stroke in a superior, then medial direction to return to the starting point.
• Repeat the entire stroke until the tissue is warm and the stones have cooled to an appropriate temperature.

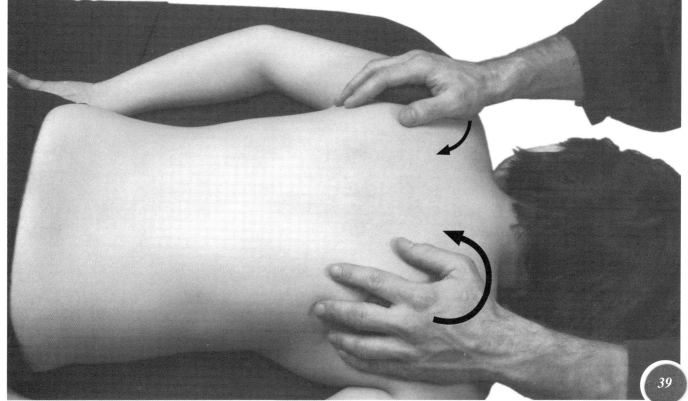

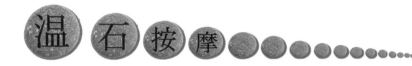

温石揉捏法
Rotation Over the Trapezius

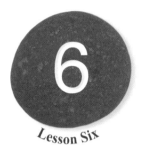

6 Lesson Six

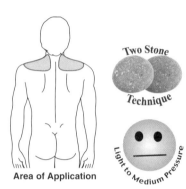

Area of Application

Two Stone Technique

Light to Medium Pressure

Modern lifestyles often create significant tension in the trapezius area. This technique is important because it releases tension in this region, which will greatly increase the effectiveness and quality of your treatment. This deep, stimulating technique follows Lesson #5 and should only be applied when your stones are at an appropriate temperature. **Do not use hot stones in this region.** If the stones are too cool, apply the previous technique with fresh stones until the temperature is appropriate. Safe and effective wrist angles are a crucial aspect of this technique, so adjust your stance and table height to facilitate proper wrist alignment. Your individually correct body position depends largely upon your height and the height of your massage table. Movement should come from your entire body and from moving your rotator cuff, instead of your wrists or other small joints. When applying this technique, keep your elbows and shoulders dropped to maintain a neutral wrist alignment and avoid hyperextension.

Step 1
- Kneel in front of the face cradle without contacting it.
- Place the stones over the trapezius, between the spine and scapula.
- Place your client's arms on the table to maximize effectiveness.

- Do not hyperextend your wrists.
- Keep your elbows and shoulders dropped and relaxed.
- Keep your torso upright, not hunched over.

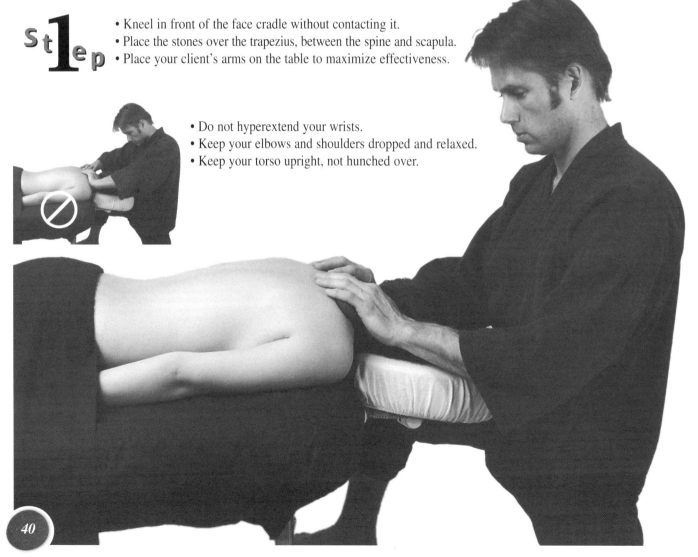

温石按摩

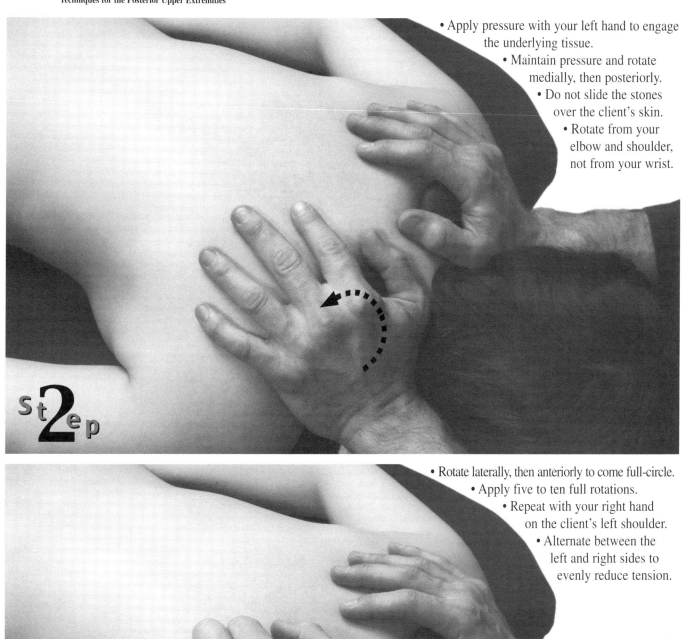

- Apply pressure with your left hand to engage the underlying tissue.
- Maintain pressure and rotate medially, then posteriorly.
- Do not slide the stones over the client's skin.
- Rotate from your elbow and shoulder, not from your wrist.

ˢᵗ2ᵉᵖ

- Rotate laterally, then anteriorly to come full-circle.
- Apply five to ten full rotations.
- Repeat with your right hand on the client's left shoulder.
- Alternate between the left and right sides to evenly reduce tension.

ˢᵗ3ᵉᵖ

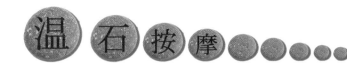

Lesson Seven

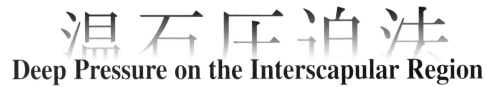

Deep Pressure on the Interscapular Region

Now that the interscapular region has been warmed by the previous techniques, it is ready for deeper stimulation. Climbing pressure is a firm application used to release deep muscle tension. People who have significant tension and problems with their neck, generally have tension in the interscapular region as well. It is important to reduce interscapular tension in order to release tension in the neck. The interscapular region, and the rhomboids in particular, often respond better when massaged and stretched in a superior direction. The amount of pressure you apply while climbing must be carefully adjusted to remain therapeutic, yet within the client's tolerance level.

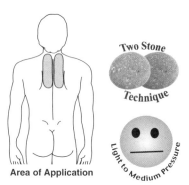

Area of Application

Two Stone Technique

Light to Medium Pressure

Step 1

- Sit or kneel in front of the face cradle.
- Grasp the stones and turn the ulna side down.
- Place the stones on either side of T-3, over the rhomboids.

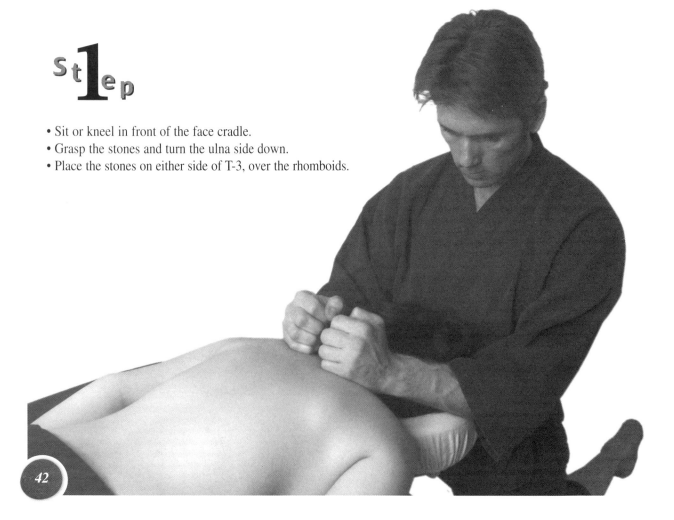

温石按摩

Step 2
• Reposition your right hand one vertebrae inferior and engage the underlying tissue.
• Maintain pressure and pull the underlying tissue superiorly.
• Tissue in this area should naturally move about one inch superior.
• Do not slide the stones over the skin or force the underlying tissue too far superior.

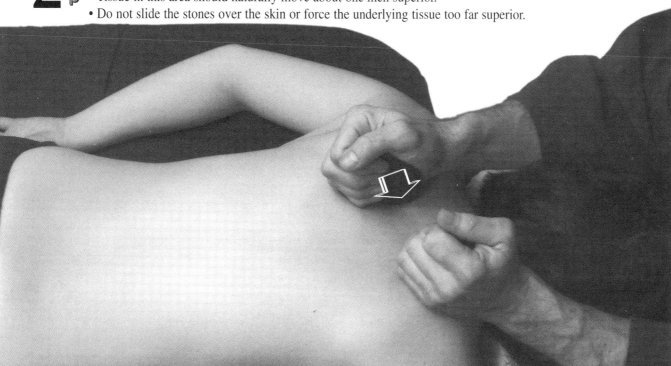

Step 3
• Reposition your left hand inferiorly, engage the underlying tissue and release pressure with your right hand.
• Maintain pressure with your left hand and pull the tissue superiorly.
• Alternate in a continuous climbing motion, until you reach the inferior angle of the scapula.
• Return to the starting position and repeat several times as desired.

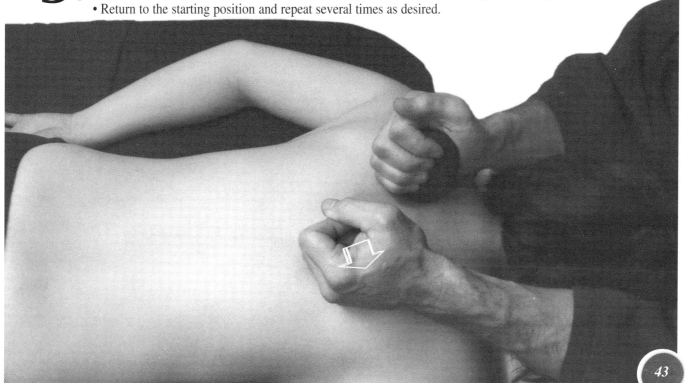

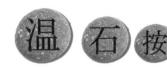

8

Lesson Eight

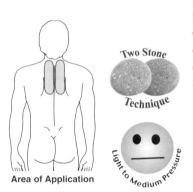

Area of Application

Two Stone Technique

Light to Medium Pressure

温石揉提法
Pivot Rotation on the Interscapular Region

There are many Bladder meridian tsubo located in the interscapular region that help reduce tension in this region. These points also reduce neck and shoulder tension and increase mobility. Tsubo in this region are often very sensitive, so you must avoid overstimulation, which can be counterproductive. If one side of the interscapular region is extremely painful, focus your treatment on tsubo located on the opposite side of the body. Treating the less painful side will help both sides release with minimal discomfort, while making the painful side more accessible. Tension and pain around interscapular tsubo often indicate lung related problems, excessive stress or problems with the neck and shoulders.

St**1**ep

- Sit or kneel by the face cradle.
- Grip the stones in both hands and place them on the inferior edge of the interscapular region.
- Drop your elbows to avoid wrist hyperextension.

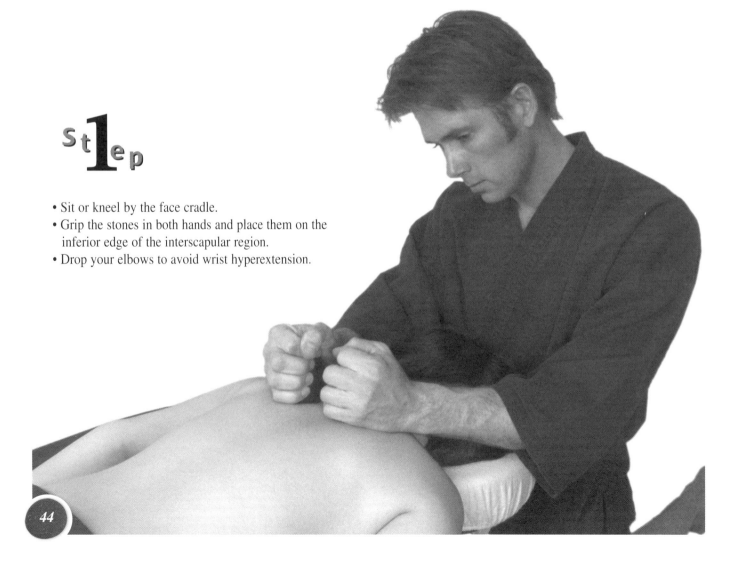

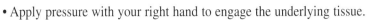

温石按摩

Step 2
- Apply pressure with your right hand to engage the underlying tissue.
- Rotate using the protruding tip of the stone as a pivot.

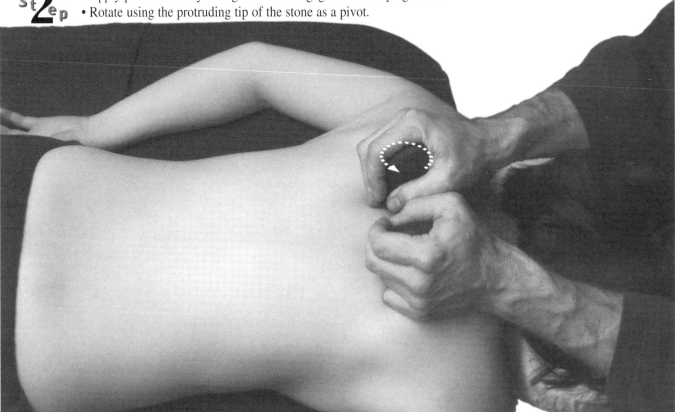

Step 3
- After three to five rotations, repeat the procedure with your left hand.
- Move both hands one vertebrae superior and repeat until you reach T1-T2.

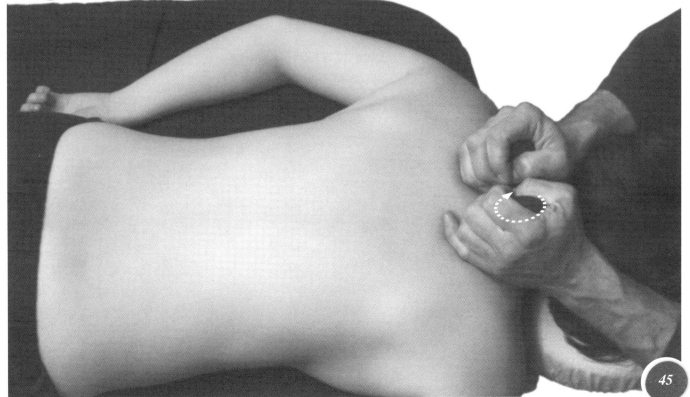

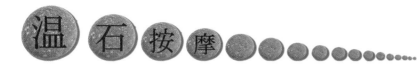

温 石 按 摩

温石圧迫法
Gentle Compression on the Posterior Neck

9

Lesson Nine

Area of Application

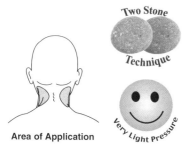

Two Stone Technique

Very Light Pressure

The neck often carries significant tension. This gentle compression technique helps alleviate some neck tension; however, neck tension will not completely release until interscapular tension has been addressed. You must properly warm the interscapular region before working on the cervicals. The neck is more fragile than other regions of the body, so you must apply this technique with caution. Place the stones carefully and only use them to stimulate the posterior cervical muscles. If you place the stones too far anterior, they will create a choking sensation for the client. Downward pressure applied into the face cradle will create discomfort on the anterior cervical and should also be avoided. To minimize wrist stress, sit as close to the face cradle as possible; however, do not allow your chest region to contact the client. Lower your body position by sitting or kneeling near the client, and drop your elbows to minimize wrist stress. Ensure that your back remains straight throughout the treatment. The neck can be very sensitive to significant temperatures, so only use stones that have cooled properly. For clients with previous neck injuries, such as whiplash or neck surgery, apply gentle pressure without rotation. In the case of severe neck problems, avoid this procedure to ensure the safety of your client.

Step 1

- Kneel or sit directly in front of the face cradle.
- Hold the stones in your lower palms.
- Place both stones over the posterior neck.
- Gently overlap your fingers and relax your elbows.

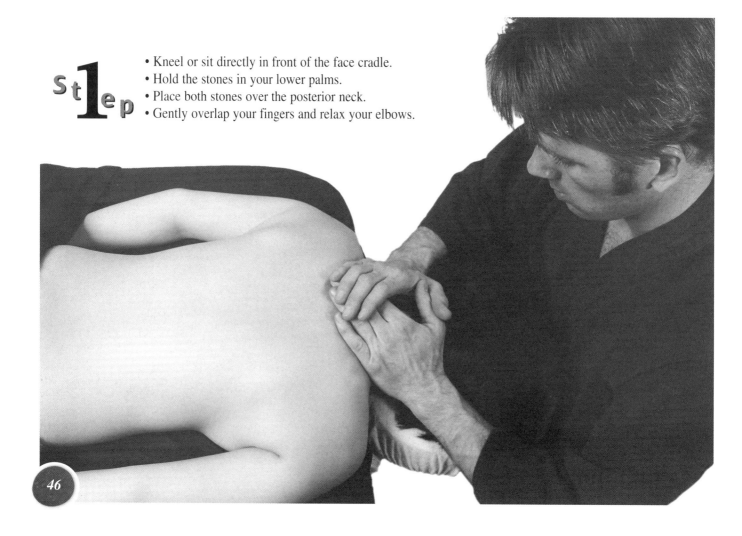

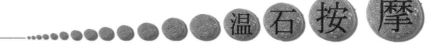

温石按摩

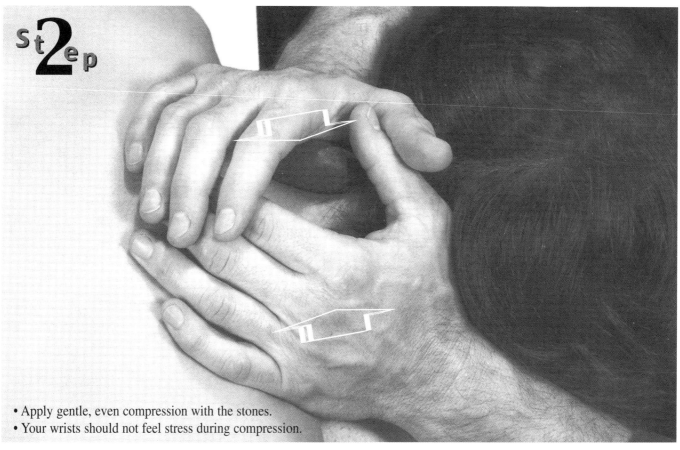

st2ep

- Apply gentle, even compression with the stones.
- Your wrists should not feel stress during compression.

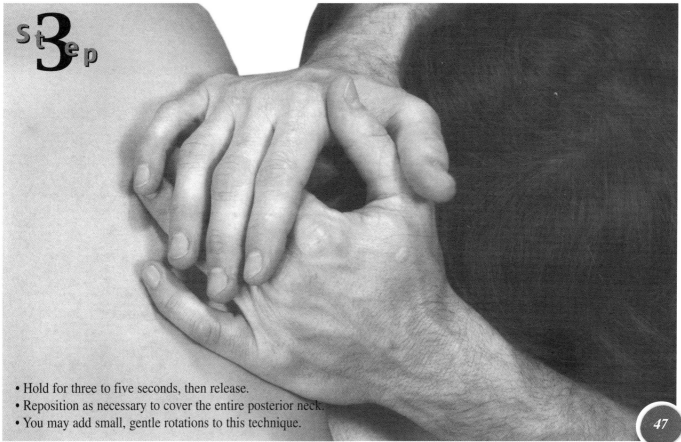

st3ep

- Hold for three to five seconds, then release.
- Reposition as necessary to cover the entire posterior neck.
- You may add small, gentle rotations to this technique.

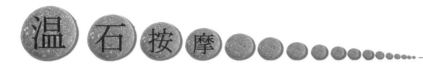

温石揉捏法
Pivot Rotation on the Occipital Ridge

10
Lesson Ten

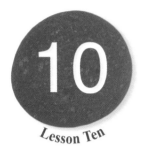

Area of Application

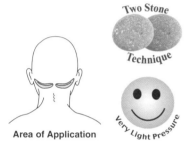
Two Stone Technique

Very Light Pressure

This pivot rotation technique was previously introduced for the interscapular region. During pivot rotations, the entire stone rotates, except for the pivot point. When using this technique on the occipital ridge, you must carefully apply rotation to avoid contacting the skull. Adjust your pressure to maintain a therapeutic level; however, keep in mind that excessive pressure can create discomfort or headaches. Before applying this technique, use the previous technique to ensure that the neck is warm. The stones should be at their coolest working temperature when applying pivot rotation on the occipital ridge. Apply this technique with the sides of the stones (as opposed to flat edges) in order to properly fit them into the occipital ridge, which is slightly inferior to the occipital bone. This is one of the most tense places in the entire neck region, so never overstimulate this area or use force to release tension. Overstimulation can be counterproductive and may even cause injury.

Step 1

- Maintain the body position from the previous technique.
- Place both stones on the occipital ridge and cup them loosely them with your hands.

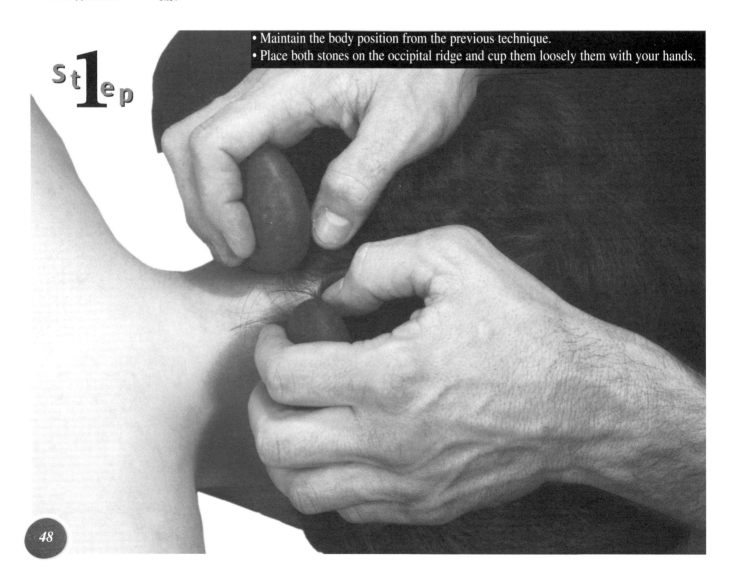

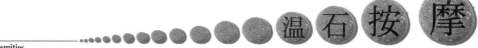

s^t**2**_{ep}
- Gently rotate your right hand, using the tip of the stone as a pivot.
- After three to five rotations, repeat with your left hand.

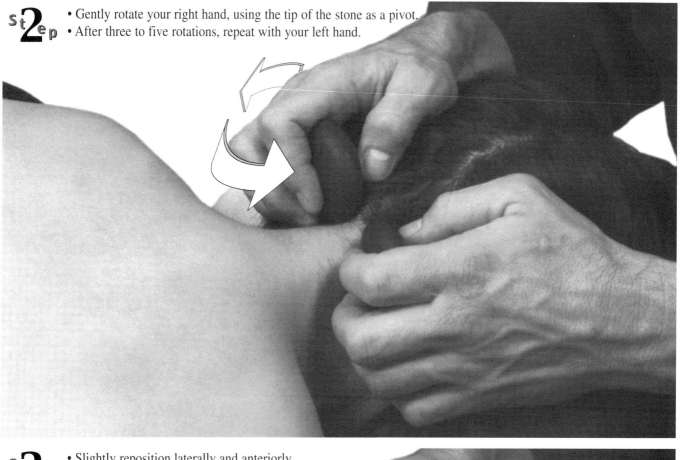

s^t**3**_{ep}
- Slightly reposition laterally and anteriorly.
- Reduce pressure as you reach the mastoid region.
- Repeat to cover the entire occipital ridge.

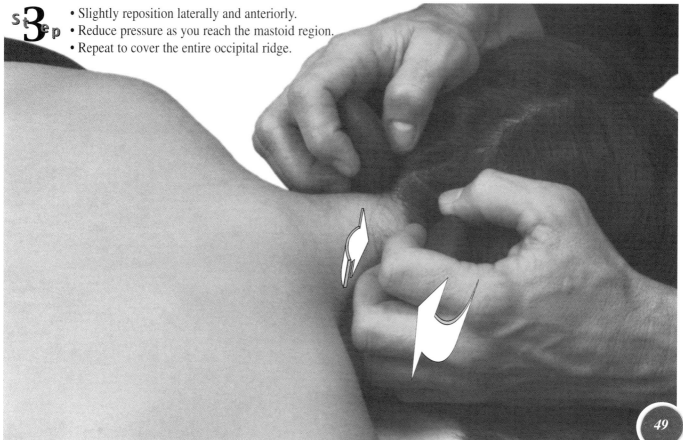

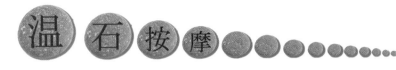

温石軽擦法
Stroking the Lateral Torso

Lesson Eleven

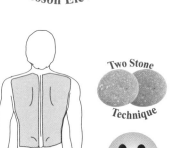

Area of Application

Two Stone Technique

Very Light Pressure

The next four lessons demonstrate techniques for the right torso and shoulder. After practicing Lessons #11-14 on the right side of the body, try them on the left side, taking care to use proper body mechanics. Apply this treatment from the shoulder girdle to the iliac crest with a fresh set of stones. Before deeply stimulating the rotator cuff, warm the lateral torso muscles to drain toxins released by earlier work into the circulatory system for elimination. This long stroke over the lateral torso warms the tissue and is used as a transition between regions. Proper posture and stance are critical for performing a smooth stroke over the entire length of the torso. Contour your hands over bony surfaces of the shoulder, scapula and iliac crest, and never contact the spinous process. When applying two-stone techniques, maintain an even, comfortable pace to prevent meridian overstimulation.

Step 1

- Stand at the head of table in front of the right shoulder.
- Place your right hand with stone at interscapular region.
- Place your left hand with stone at the lateral scapula.
- Lower your stance and shoulders to maintain proper wrist alignment.

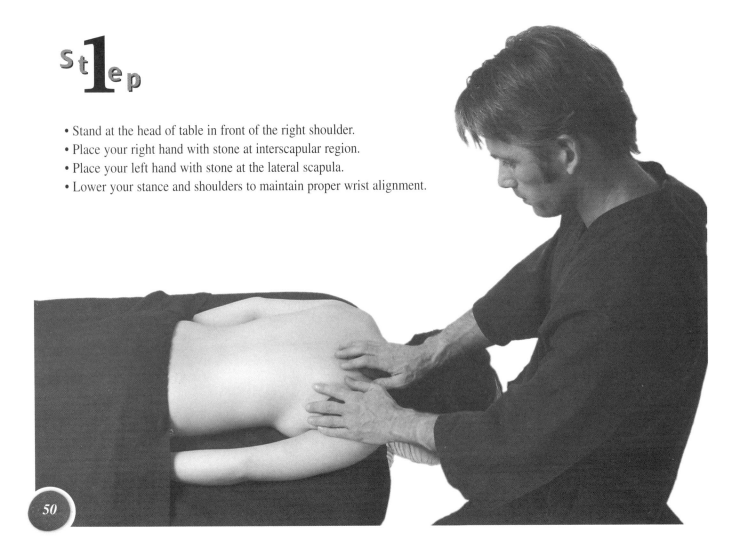

温石按摩

Step 2
- Stroke inferiorly along the lateral torso with both hands simultaneously.
- Do not contact the spinal process with the right stone.

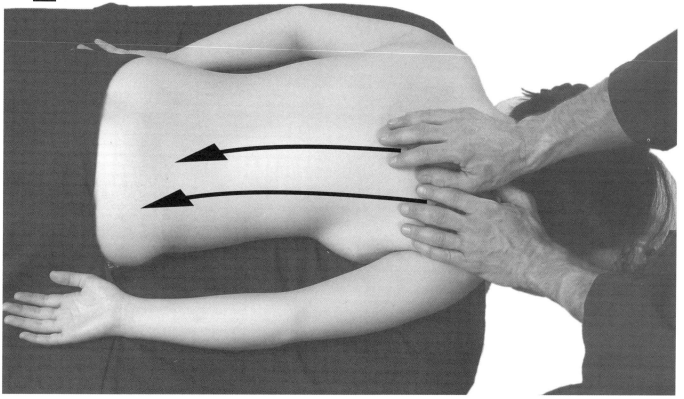

Step 3
- Stoke until you reach the gluteal region.
- Reverse your stroke along the same path.
- Repeat five to seven sets.

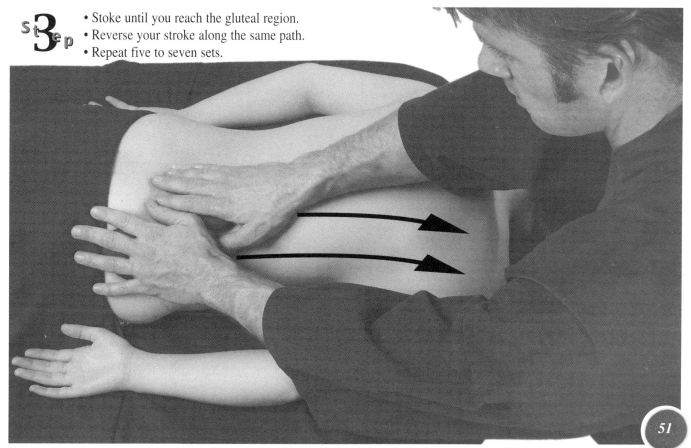

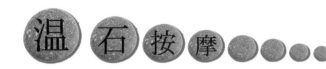

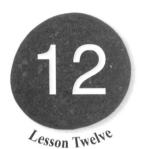

Lesson Twelve

温石軽擦法

Stroking the Posterior Shoulder and Arm

Continue warming the upper arm and shoulder region with this light stroke over the posterior shoulder. This stroke focuses on the area from the upper arm to the rotator cuff, which follows the direction of *ki* flow to three meridians: Large Intestine, Triple Heater and Small Intestine. The return stroke is lighter and is only used to retain heat in the tissue. Use caution near bony surfaces by maintaining a hand position that will ensure your ability to contour. The first stroke (Steps 2 & 3) focuses on the Large Intestine and Triple Heater meridians, while the second stroke (Steps 4 & 5) focuses on the Triple Heater and Small Intestine meridians.

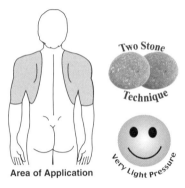

Area of Application

Two Stone
Technique

Very Light Pressure

Step 1

- Gently lift and hang your client's arm off the side of the table.
- Place hands with stones by the elbow on the posterior arm.

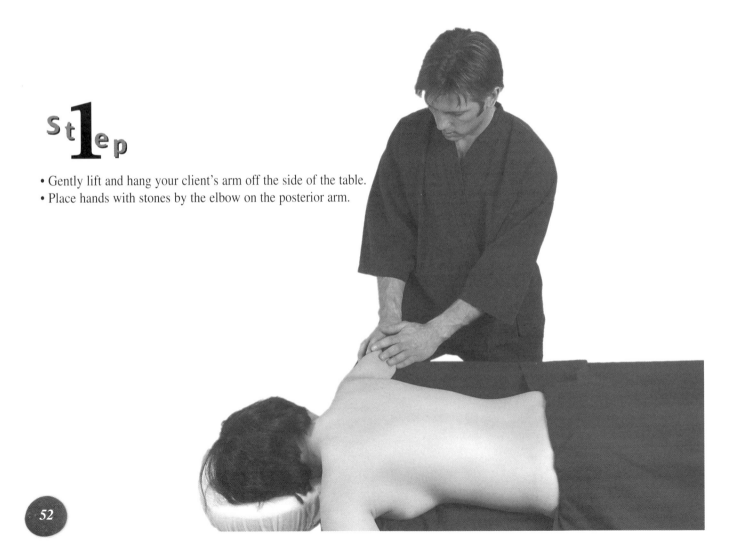

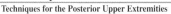

温 石 按 摩

Step 2
- Stroke medially along the arm with both hands.
- Stroke using entire body movement.

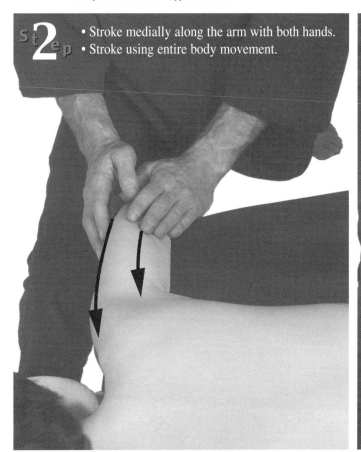

Step 3
- End the stroke over the shoulder.
- Reverse the stroke toward the elbow.
- Repeat three to five times.

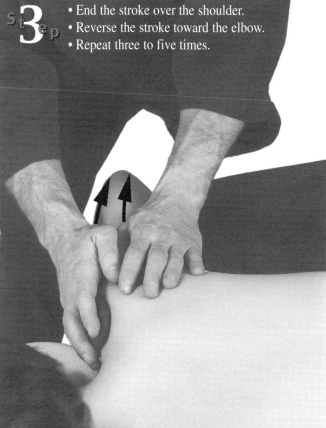

Step 4
- Stroke toward the shoulder blade.
- Stroke slightly inferior to Step 2.

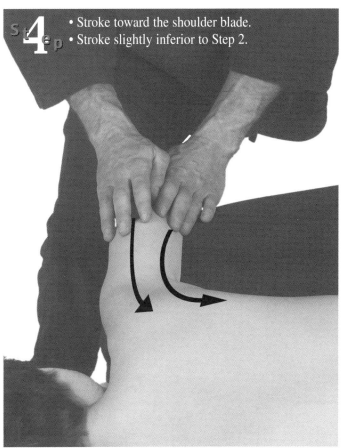

Step 5
- End the stroke over the scapula.
- Reverse direction and repeat the procedure.

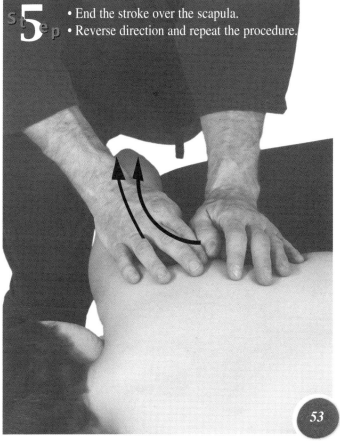

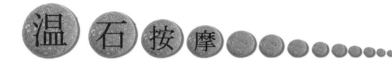

温石揉提法

Rotation on the Axillary Region with Two Stones

Lesson Thirteen

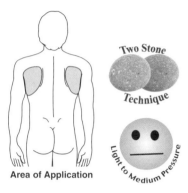

Area of Application

Two Stone Technique

Light to Medium Pressure

After warming the arm and shoulder region with the previous techniques, this two-stone rotation will reduce muscle tension in the axillary region. The infraspinatus and teres muscles can be very tense. People with occupations that require repetitive hand and arm movement, such as typists, hair dressers and massage therapists, will experience a higher degree of tension in this area. These three muscles are crucial for upper torso alignment and if they harbor tension, the rhomboid muscle will also become tense. When the rhomboid becomes tense, neck mobility decreases. Tension in the infraspinatus and teres muscles also effects the pectoralis muscles. When the pectoralis muscles are tense, they restrict lung movement, which can lead to fatigue or emotional depression. You can apply this technique while standing, kneeling or sitting in a chair; however, for taller therapists, kneeling may be safer for the wrists. Although you may sit in a chair to apply this technique, sitting in a chair with wheels may not provide the stability necessary for the stroke.

St**1**ep

- Stand or kneel at the side of the table near the arm.
- Place both hands with stones over the axillary region.

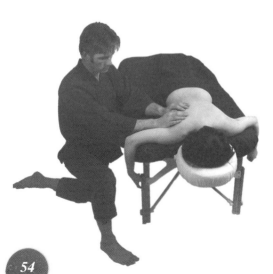

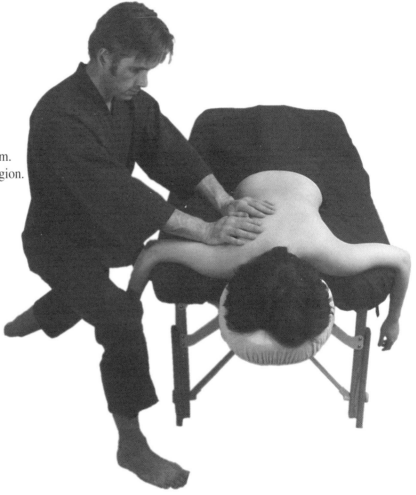

温石按摩

Step 2
- Apply pressure to engage the underlying tissue.
- Rotate in a superior to medial direction.
- Use your fingertips as a pivot for the rotation.

Step 3
- Continue rotating inferiorly, then laterally.
- Repeat three to five times.

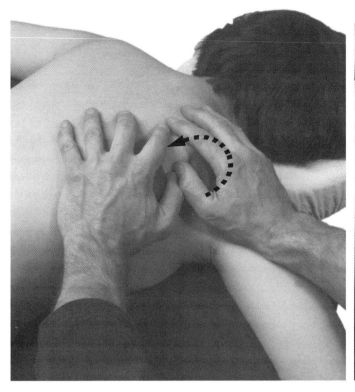

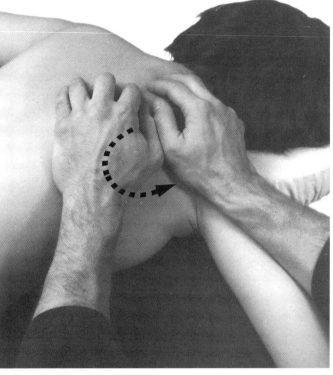

Step 4
- Reposition inferiorly and repeat the rotation.

Step 5
- Continue repositing to address the entire region.

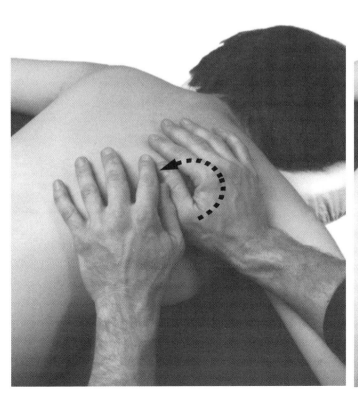

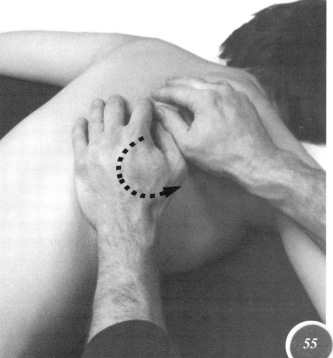

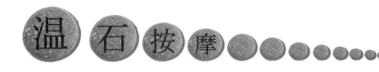

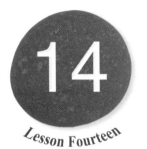

温石揉捏法
Rotation on the Infraspinatus and Teres

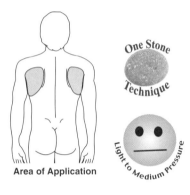

Area of Application

One Stone Technique

Light to Medium Pressure

This technique is a continuation of the previous technique; however, this rotation delivers more stimulation. The technique used in this lesson is applied at a therapeutic level and may not be suitable for all clients. Sufficiently warm the region with the previous techniques before applying this lesson. Due to the location and intensity of this rotation, you must be careful not to overwork specific muscle attachments. Do not introduce new stones before this technique, because this area is extremely sensitive to high temperatures. If you must introduce new stones at this point, repeat Lessons #11 and 12 until the stones are cool enough for this rotation. Like Lesson #13, we recommend that you apply this treatment from a kneeling or seated position. This position ensures that your wrist angle remains low and permits more direct contact with the lateral scapula. Raise the client's arm and extend it across your knee to slightly stretch the infraspinatus and teres muscles. Stretching this muscle makes this technique more effective, and requires less effort. Treating a relaxed muscle requires more pressure and effort. As the infraspinatus and teres muscles release, and shoulder flexibility increases, you may need to further elevate the arm to sustain a therapeutic level. You may also continue this technique over the latissimus dorsi to increase effectiveness. This is a one-stone technique.

Step 1

• Sit or kneel at the corner of the table.
• Rest the client's arm over your right knee.
• Stabilize their arm with your right hand.
• Place your left hand with stone over the infraspinatus.

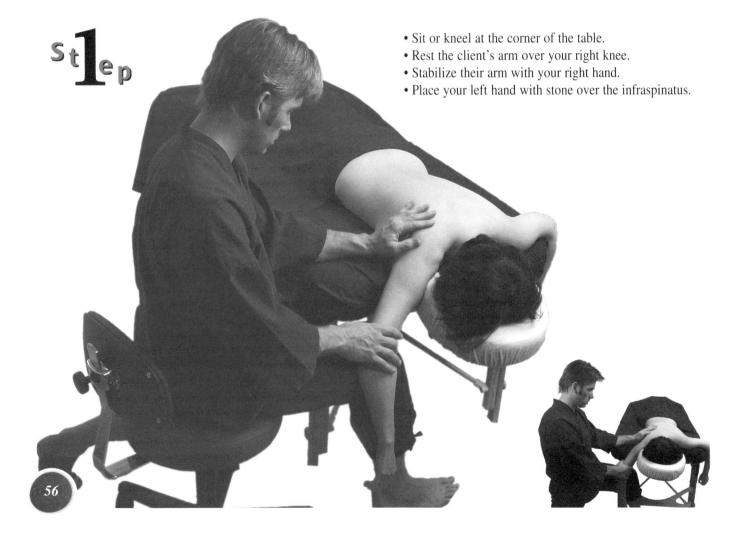

温石按摩

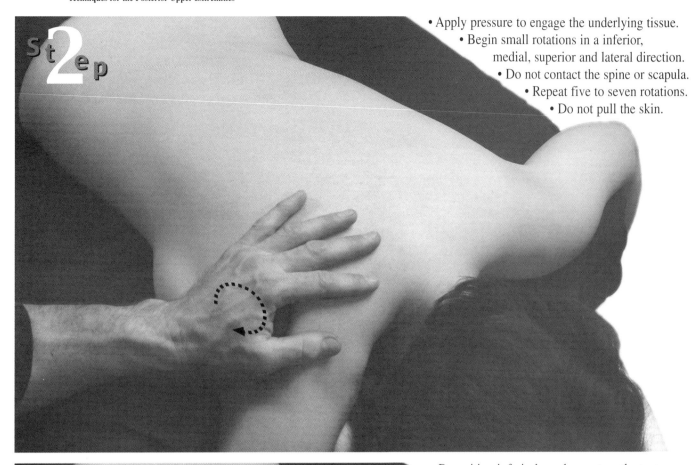

- Apply pressure to engage the underlying tissue.
- Begin small rotations in a inferior, medial, superior and lateral direction.
- Do not contact the spine or scapula.
- Repeat five to seven rotations.
- Do not pull the skin.

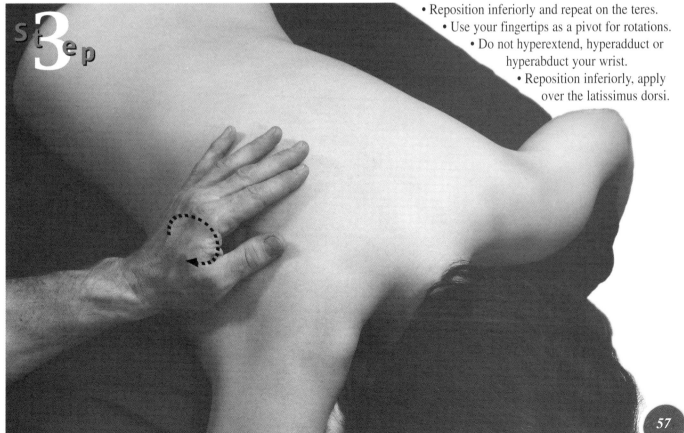

- Reposition inferiorly and repeat on the teres.
- Use your fingertips as a pivot for rotations.
- Do not hyperextend, hyperadduct or hyperabduct your wrist.
- Reposition inferiorly, apply over the latissimus dorsi.

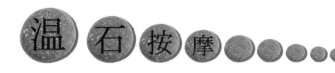

15

Lesson Fifteen

温石軽擦法
Cross-Stroking on the Lumbar Region

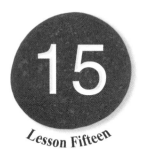

Area of Application

Two Stone
Technique

Very Light Pressure

This is the initial warming stroke for the low back region. The range of this stroke includes the lumbar and lower thoracic areas, as well as the lateral torso. Due to the size of these areas, full body movements are necessary to efficiently perform this technique. Your stance should be relatively wide and your feet should be perpendicular to stabilize your body movements. This stroke is achieved by coordinating arm and hip movement. Using arm movement alone will stress the posterior thoracic muscles and restrict low back movement. Your pelvis must move freely to accommodate arm movement. Adjust the height of your stance to keep your wrists in a horizontal plane, which allows you to safely contour the hips during this stroke. If you are unable to contour bony surfaces, you may need to avoid those areas. This technique uses the weight of your hands on the stones, rather than strength, to apply pressure.

Step 1

• Stand in a wide stance by the lower back and face the table.
• Place hands with stones on either side of the lateral lumbar.
• Lower your stance to maintain a proper wrist angle.

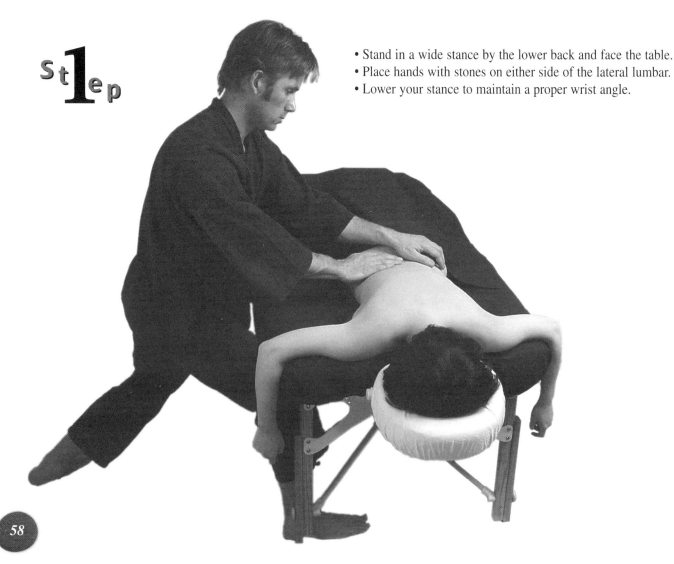

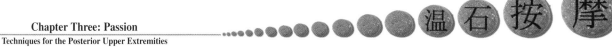

温石按摩

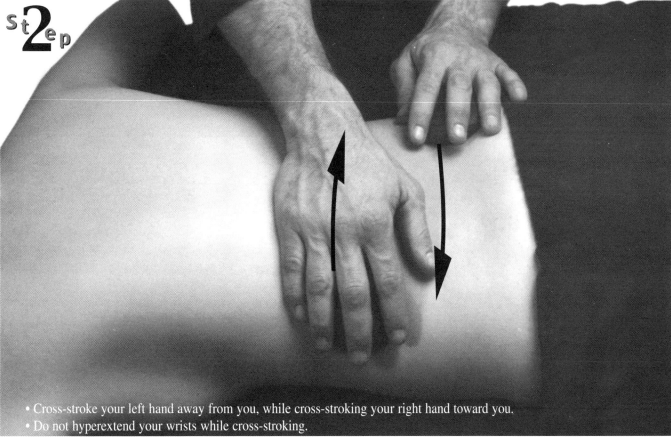

st2ep

- Cross-stroke your left hand away from you, while cross-stroking your right hand toward you.
- Do not hyperextend your wrists while cross-stroking.

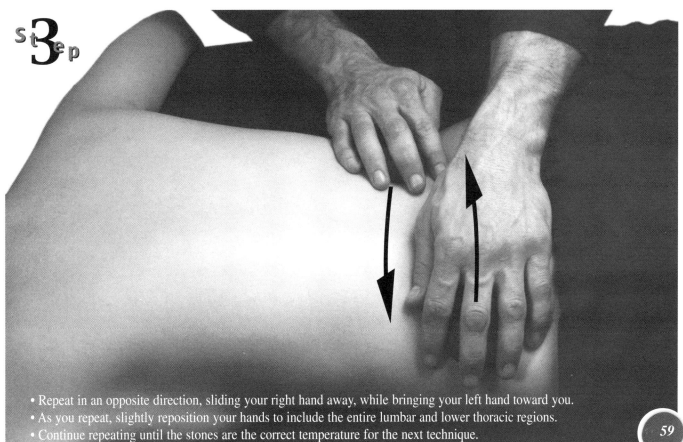

st3ep

- Repeat in an opposite direction, sliding your right hand away, while bringing your left hand toward you.
- As you repeat, slightly reposition your hands to include the entire lumbar and lower thoracic regions.
- Continue repeating until the stones are the correct temperature for the next technique.

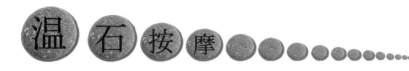

温石軽擦法
Stroking the Low Back

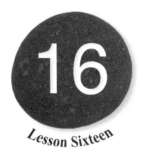

Lesson Sixteen

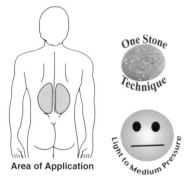

Area of Application

One Stone Technique

Light to Medium Pressure

After warming the low back with the previous lesson, combine this slow, deep stroke with a gentle stretch to release tight erector and quadratus lumborum muscles. To achieve the low back erector stretch necessary for this stroke, anchor the hip by placing your hand over the sacro-iliac joint. Limit hand and wrist tension, by hooking the stone between your thenar eminence and the quadratus lumborum, while keeping your hand and fingers relaxed. Gripping the stone creates unnecessary tension in the hand, forearm and elbow. Keep your hand in line with your forearm, and your elbow relaxed to ensure uninterrupted *ki* flow through the wrist and prevent hyperabduction. When performing deep strokes, it is most effective to use your entire body during application. Keeping your hands, wrists and shoulders relaxed will project relaxation upon the client's body; conversely, they will also register your muscle tension. Understanding this concept is the key to giving many effective massages over a long period of time. If you feel stress in your joints, evaluate the following: the position of the stones, your body mechanics and the client's resistance to the intensity of pressure. In this stroke, proper traction between the stone and the skin is very important. Without proper glide, you may pull your client's skin and deeper tissue. If you have too much glide, this technique is less therapeutic.

St**1**ep

• Stand by the client's hip with your thighs against the massage table.
• Place your left hand on the iliac crest.
• Place your right hand with stone over the lumbar on the erector muscle.

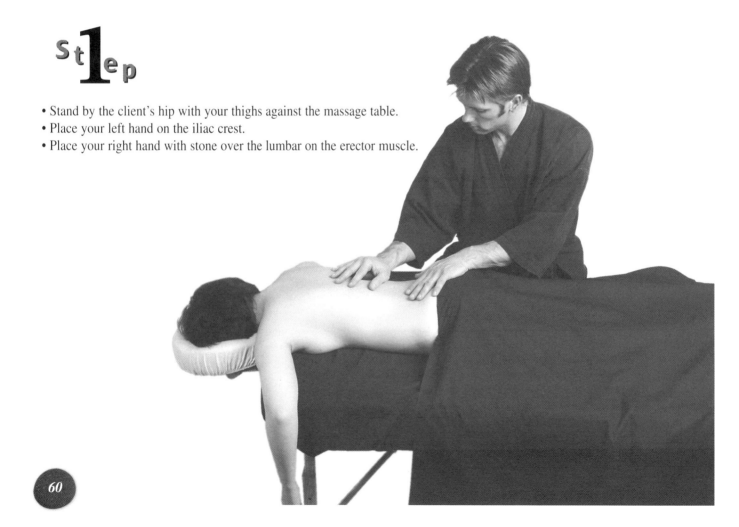

温 石 按 摩

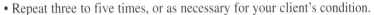

Step 2

- Stabilize the tissue with your left hand and place your right hand slightly superior to the iliac crest.
- Engage the underlying tissue and stroke superiorly, while maintaining firm pressure.
- Stroke on the erector muscles, parallel to the spine, but do not contact the spinal process.

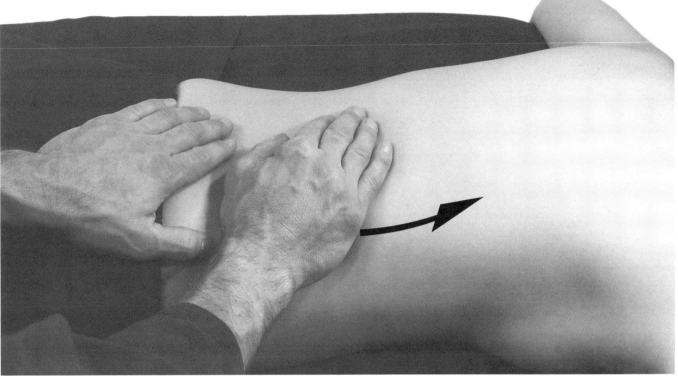

Step 3

- When you reach the rib cage, stroke back to the starting position with light pressure.
- Use body movement for this stroke and drop your elbows to maintain a safe wrist angle.
- Repeat three to five times, or as necessary for your client's condition.

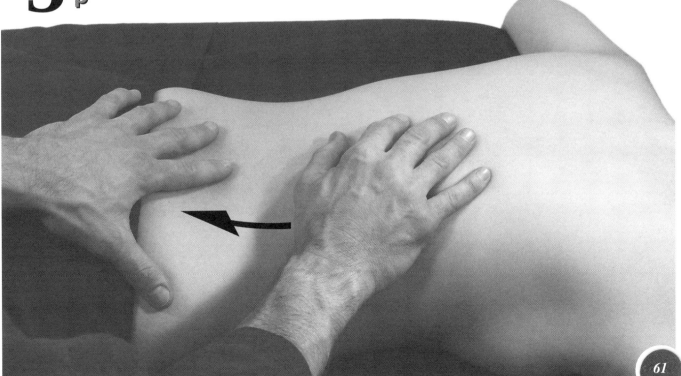

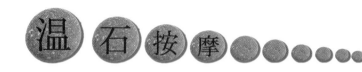

温石揉提法
Rotation on the Low Back

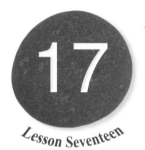

Lesson Seventeen

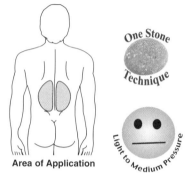

Area of Application

One Stone Technique

Light to Medium Pressure

Rotation is the primary technique for working the back in traditional Japanese massage. In anma, rotation actually incorporates kneading movements. This technique is the foundation of anma, and is one of the most difficult techniques to master. When applied with inadequate pressure, this technique is not therapeutic. When applied with excessive pressure, the client resists, making the technique counterproductive, and therefore, an inefficient use of your time. To properly apply this technique, keep your elbow, shoulder and arm loose. Rotation comes from your elbow and shoulder, not from your wrist. Applying pressure with a misaligned wrist is harmful for you and less effective for your client. To address the varying layers of the erector muscles, adjust the height of your stance to keep your arm on a horizontal plane. This position allows you to isolate areas that require specific attention. The true art of anma massage is understanding that the more relaxed your are, the more therapeutic your treatment will be. When you are relaxed, you can adapt to subtle changes in your client's *ki* flow and muscle condition; otherwise, your tension may inhibit *ki* flow communication.

Step 1

- Maintain the body position from the previous technique.
- Apply pressure with your right hand to engage the underlying tissue at the lateral edge of the erector muscle, inferior to the rib cage.
- Stabilize the pelvis with your left hand.

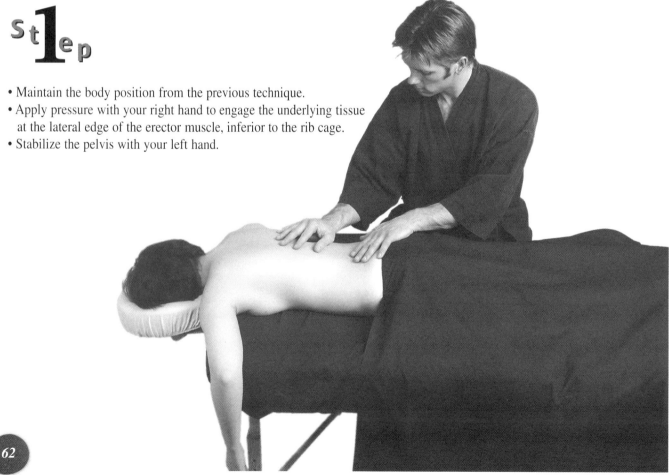

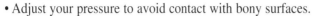 温石按摩

Step 2

- Rotate your right hand in a superior, medial, inferior and lateral direction.
- Apply pressure during the superior-medial rotation and ease pressure during the inferior-lateral rotation.
- Adjust your pressure to avoid contact with bony surfaces.

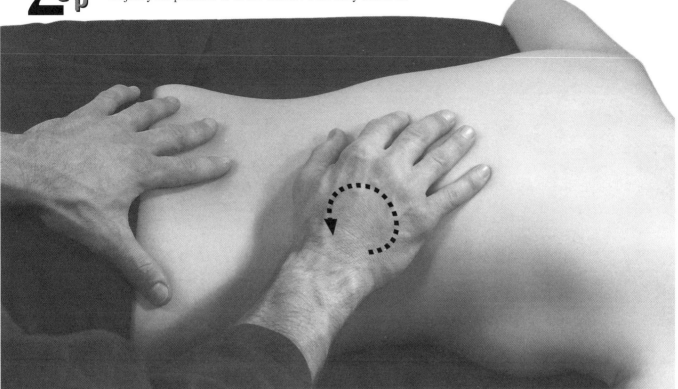

Step 3

- Apply three to five rotations, then move half a palm-width inferior and repeat.
- Continue repositioning and repeat until your right hand reaches the iliac crest.
- Drop your elbows to avoid hyperabduction, hyperadduction or hyperextension.
- Repeat this entire procedure two to three times as necessary.

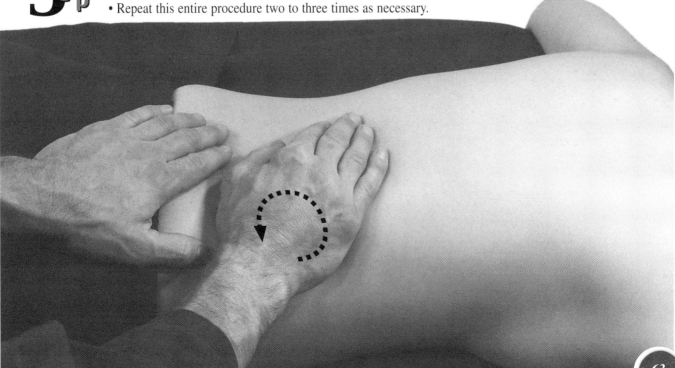

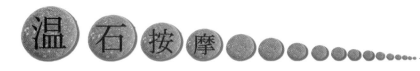

Lesson Eighteen

Pivot Rotation on the Iliac Crest Attachment

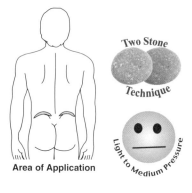

Area of Application

Two Stone Technique

Light to Medium Pressure

This technique is suitable for all posterior attachments of the iliac crest, quadratus lumborum, obliques and erector spinae muscles. This technique relieves low back tension and focuses primarily on the quadratus lumborum, which is the key to releasing low back tension. This technique works very well for clients with disabling low back tension, but is not recommended for more serious low back conditions, such as ruptured or herniated discs and sprained lumbar ligaments. If you receive any indication that your pressure is too deep, either verbal or non-verbal, re-evaluate the depth of your pressure or the client's condition. Overworking this area is contraindicated, because it creates latent inflammation and compounds the problem. When applying this technique, a certain amount of pressure is necessary for the treatment to be therapeutic. If a release does not occur, you must first address tension in another area of the body. Overworking the low back will not solve the problem until the primary tension is released. When applying this technique, use both stones together as a single unit. This is a deep pivot, not a deep grinding technique. The pivot point on the muscle is created by a larger rotation from your hands. Use the edge of the stone to engage the muscle attachment, then begin slow rotations. Slow rotation gives the nervous system adequate time to re-educate the muscle.

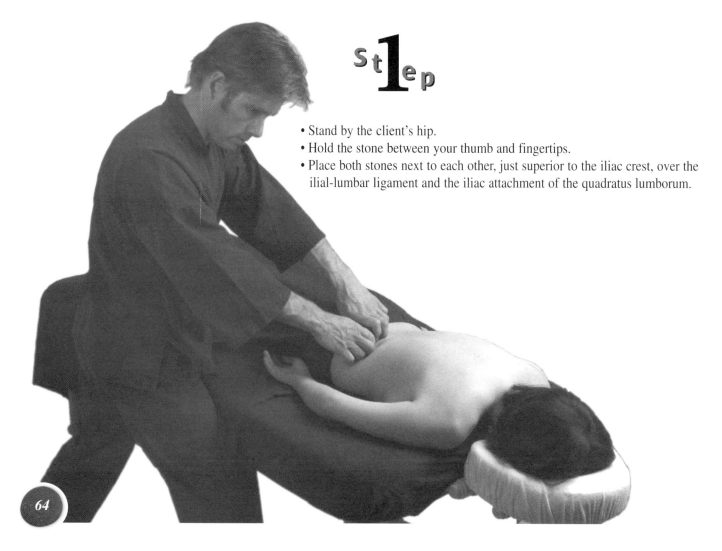

Step 1

- Stand by the client's hip.
- Hold the stone between your thumb and fingertips.
- Place both stones next to each other, just superior to the iliac crest, over the ilial-lumbar ligament and the iliac attachment of the quadratus lumborum.

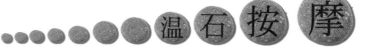

温石按摩

- Apply downward pressure to engage the underlying tissue.
- Use the edge of the stone as a pivot, and rotate in a medial, then superior direction.
- Do not apply pressure to the lumbar vertebrae or the iliac crest.

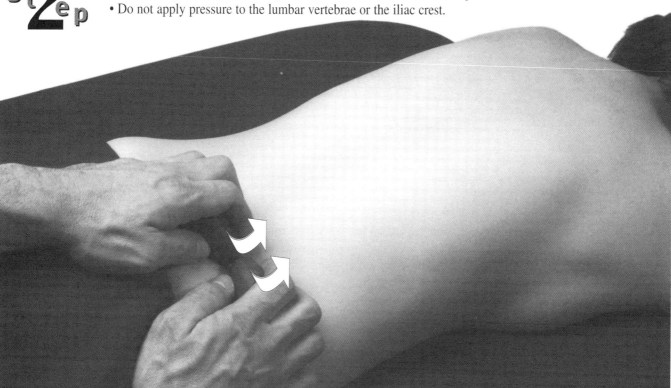

st**3**ep

- Continue in a lateral and inferior direction to complete the rotation.
- Repeat the rotation eight to ten times.
- Do not pull or glide over the skin.

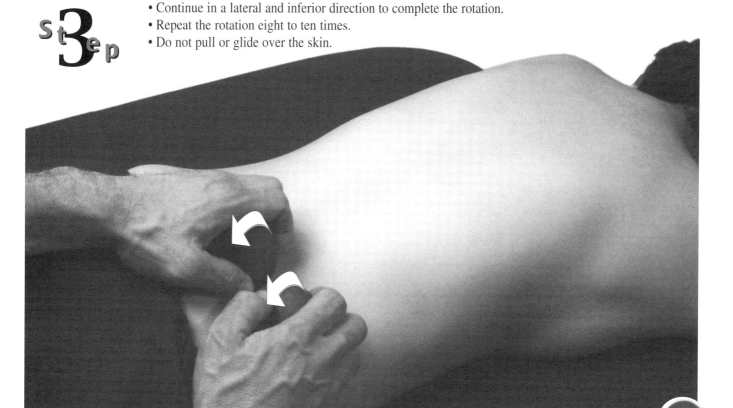

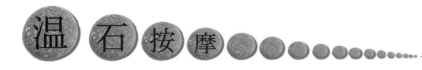

Lesson Nineteen

温石揉提法
Rotation at the Upper Gluteal Region

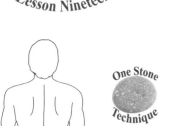

Area of Application

One Stone Technique

Light to Medium Pressure

Many people carry tension in their hips, but the majority of people are unaware of it until they receive bodywork. This technique reduces hip tension, in order to alleviate low back stress. This technique uses anma rotation on the glutes, but also requires that you stabilize the low back. Stabilizing the low back provides a gentle stretch above and below the iliac crest. This technique is problematic, because you run the risk of hyperabducting or hyperextending your wrists. We strongly emphasize proper wrist angle to prevent potential problems before they occur. To properly apply this technique, you must deliver this stroke from a horizontal plane. If your body mechanics are too high, you will deliver downward force, which will create unnecessary pressure on your wrists. If there is low back restriction, such as a pre-existing low back injury, this technique may aggravate that condition. In this case, treatment can still occur by stabilizing the pelvis to minimize low back movement, but only if the low back condition is not acute. This is a one-stone technique and should be applied with small rotations to avoid wrist strain, especially when working on larger individuals. While performing this technique on the gluteals, the fingertips of your working hand must remain on the lateral side of the gluteal region to ensure the modesty of your client.

Step 1

- Stand at the head of the table in front of the right shoulder.
- Place your left hand with stone on the upper gluteus.
- Place your right hand on the right side of the lower back for stability.

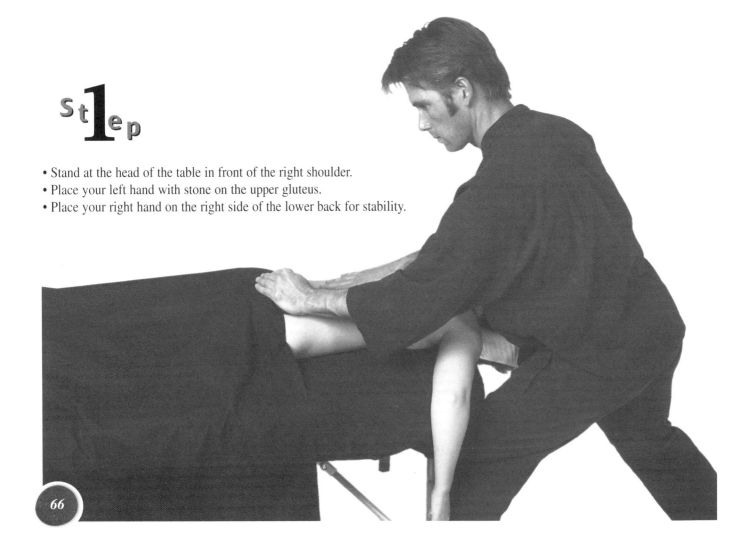

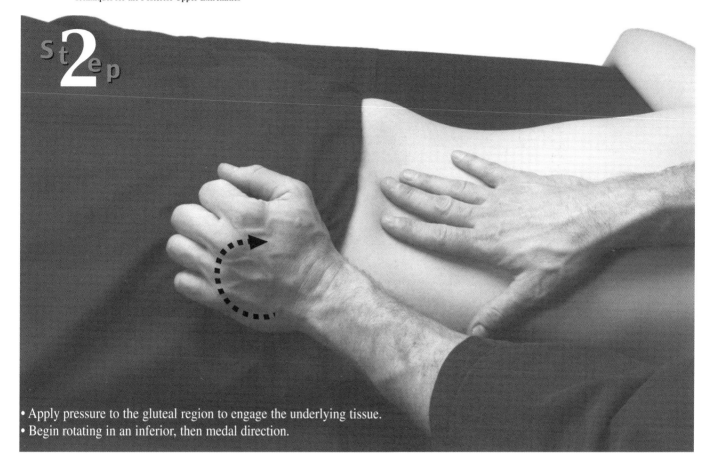

• Apply pressure to the gluteal region to engage the underlying tissue.
• Begin rotating in an inferior, then medal direction.

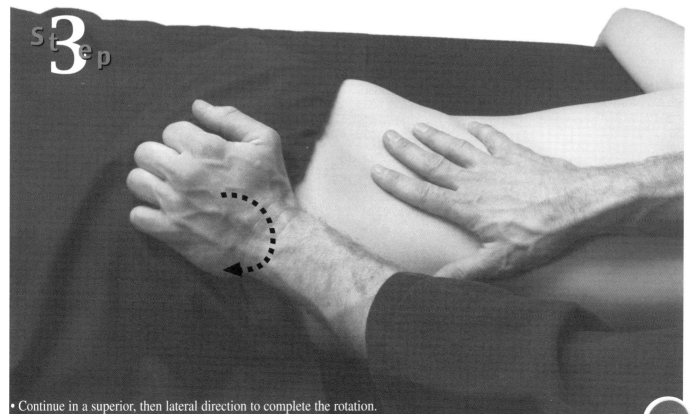

• Continue in a superior, then lateral direction to complete the rotation.
• Repeat five to seven rotations, then slightly reposition to address the upper gluteal region.

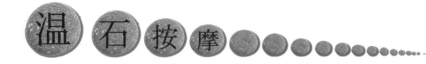

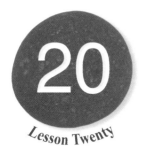

Lesson Twenty

温石軽擦法
Japanese Myofascial Release on the Low Back

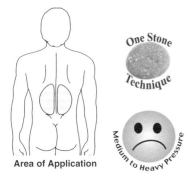

Area of Application

One Stone Technique

Medium to Heavy Pressure

We are introducing one Japanese myofascial release technique, which is believed to have been developed four to five thousand years ago. The oldest written record of this technique is from the 5th century. *Shin ken shu ho* literally translates as "to release adhered myofascial and other adhesions in the human body." This technique addresses not only fascial adhesions, but muscle to muscle, fascia to muscle, all layers of skin and other tissue, muscle to bone and other unnecessary adhesions that often create structural distortions in the human body. Ancient Japanese texts document seven dead structural centers throughout the human body where restrictive adhesions are located. This technique addresses this region of the low back. Everyday habits, such as occupational habits, sleeping habits and your existing structure, reinforce the restrictions found in these seven dead structural centers. For example, working on the computer for eight hours a day causes many people to experience tissue adhesion in the upper back, resulting in limited mobility. Limited mobility creates even more adhesion, which begins a terrible cycle. This myofascial technique is one of the most difficult, because not only is it hard to master, it is extremely hard on your fingers if performed incorrectly. Working with warm stones makes it easier to release adhesions and is slightly less stressful for your hands. This example is one of the most effective myofascial techniques for the lower back. Mastering this traditional Japanese technique requires that you go beyond the mastery of traditional massage techniques. Accomplishing structure mobility is easy, but unless you have a complete understanding of the alignment between the feet, legs and pelvis, stabilizing the structure and reducing adhesions will be difficult.

Step 1

- Stand in a stable stance by the client's right hip.
- Place right hand without stone over the lower back, perpendicular to the spine, on the right side of the iliac crest.
- Place left hand with stone over the right low back erector, perpendicular to your right hand.

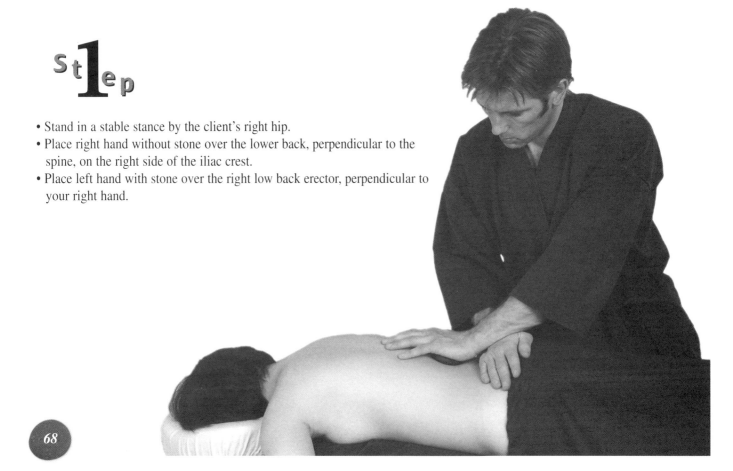

温石按摩

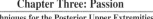

Step 2

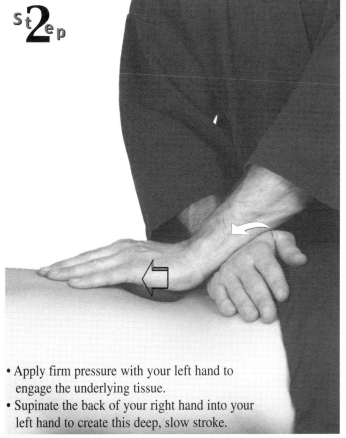

- Apply firm pressure with your left hand to engage the underlying tissue.
- Supinate the back of your right hand into your left hand to create this deep, slow stroke.

Step 3

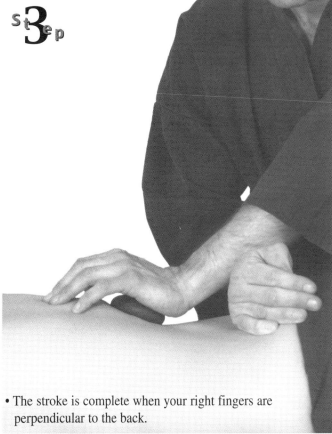

- The stroke is complete when your right fingers are perpendicular to the back.

Step 4

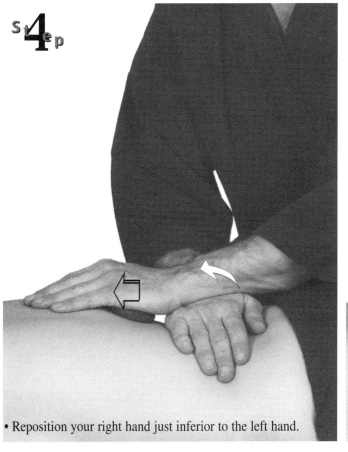

- Reposition your right hand just inferior to the left hand.

Step 5

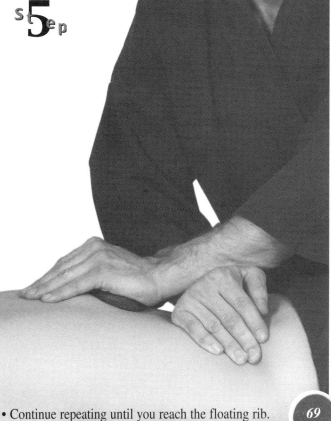

- Continue repeating until you reach the floating rib.

69

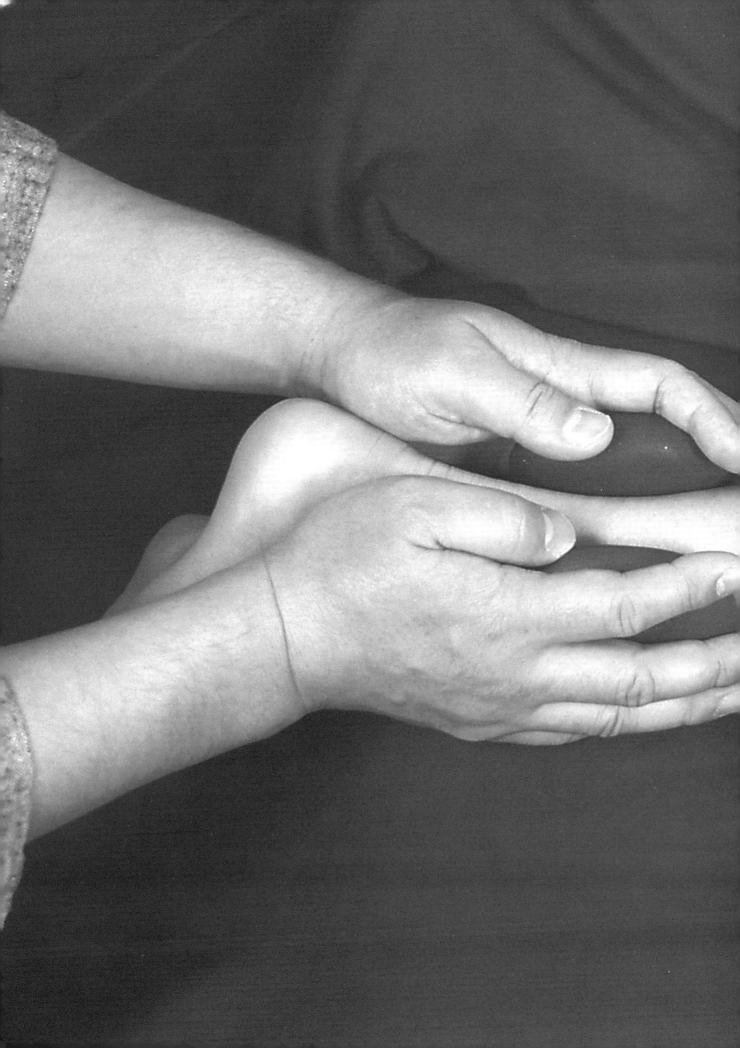

Chapter Four
REJUVENATION

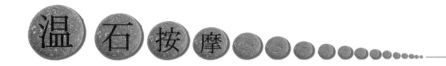

Chapter Four
REJUVENATION

Techniques for the Posterior Lower Extremities

In this chapter, we explain ten Japanese Hot Stone Massage techniques for the hips, posterior legs and feet. The second stage of this treatment represents soil. Often mistranslated as "earth," as in heaven and earth, this character represents the material soil, not the location of the earth.

The hips, legs and feet are the foundation of the human structure. Slight distortions in foot and pelvis alignment can impact the entire body. Neck and shoulder tension often repeatedly occurs until you correct foot and pelvis alignment. When a structural imbalance occurs, human energy also becomes imbalanced and the entire body experiences the imbalance throughout. Balancing tension in the legs, hips, feet and lower back is very important for returning your client's body structure to the most anatomically correct position possible.

We demonstrate these rejuvenation techniques on the right side of the body only. You should perform these techniques to completion on one side, before moving to the other side of the body. If you are working the hip or upper thigh region and the draping becomes a problem, these techniques may also be performed over the sheets. If the stones are too warm during any technique, you should perform the technique over the sheets until they have cooled appropriately. If you see an unusual foot condition, or if the feet are very moist and difficult to stroke, you may also perform foot massage techniques over the sheets.

One bolster is required at the ankles to support the lower legs. This bolster will ease low back strain and maintain relaxed muscle tone in the legs. Your stance and body mechanics are paramount to the success and safety of these treatments. Adjust your stance and lower your body to reduce wrist angle. When wrist angle is compromised, your treatment is less effective, because a higher wrist angle locks your wrists and inhibits smooth movement. Maintain smooth movement by keeping your forearms and wrists as straight as possible.

When you are more familiar with Japanese Hot Stone Massage, you can treat the low back, hip and thigh with seamless transition. For training clarification, we have divided the upper and lower extremities; however, you should seamlessly integrate treatment throughout the entire body. The upper and lower regions of the body are strongly connected, so you must treat the entire body as one single unit, rather than as isolated parts.

Not only are the posterior, lower extremities important for the human structure, three important meridians begin in the feet and run through the medial thigh. The Kidney, Spleen and Liver meridians are the three most important meridians for sustaining proper body function.

温石按摩

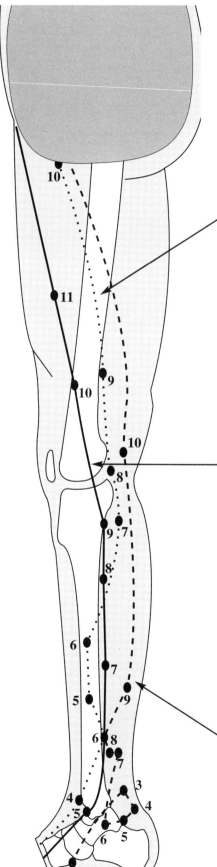

Meridians in the Medial Legs

The Kidney, Spleen and Liver meridians that run through the medial legs, are often considered to be the three most important meridians in the human body. Balancing these three meridians is essential for restoring balance in the human body. Many Japanese acupuncturists and traditional Japanese massage therapists often focus primarily on balancing these three meridians during their treatments.

Please note that when an internal organ is capitalized, it refers to the Asian form of the organ. Asian and Western ideas of internal organ function are often quite different. This book briefly introduces meridians, but for further information about meridians, tsubo and their functions, please refer to *Shiatsu for the Hand* and *Shiatsu for the Foot*.

Kidney Meridian

The East Asian understanding of the Kidneys is quite different from that of Western physiology. The East Asian concept of the Kidneys is much closer to the adrenal gland, than it is to the Western concept of the Kidneys as a filtration system. East Asian medical tradition refers to the Kidneys as the "Palace of Labor and Strength." Without the Kidneys, life cannot be sustained, because vital essence is stored within the Kidneys. Essence (*sei*) is the most elemental substance, which sustains the activity and life of the human body. *Sei* is the primary foundation of human energy and all human function. The Kidneys are responsible for supplying this essence to all internal organs. The Kidneys also store the essence received from one's parents, which contains their genetic code. Therefore, the Kidneys are also closely connected to the growth and organic development of an individual throughout life and hormonal development, including adrenal function. Healthy Kidneys are also important for brain function and strong bones.

Spleen Meridian

Western medicine doesn't consider the Spleen to be a very important organ. In East Asian medicine, however, the Spleen, along with the Kidney and Liver, is considered to be one of the most important organs for human function. In traditional East Asian medicine, the Spleen encompasses the functions of both the pancreas and the spleen, and the two are considered to be one organ. In fact, many characteristics of Spleen function are much closer to that of the Pancreas, than the Spleen itself. The Spleen's main function is to distribute nutrients throughout the body. Nutrients are carried within liquids, mainly blood, and the Spleen distributes the nutrients and blood together. If the Spleen is malfunctioning, the body will not receive the necessary amount of food essence and *ki*. One of the Spleen's most important jobs is conditioning the blood and keeping the blood within the vessels. The blood distributes nutrients to all parts of the body. When blood is not flowing correctly throughout the body, the muscles do not receive enough nutrients; therefore, they become achy and lose both mass and strength. The hydration, shape, gloss and color of the lips generally indicates Spleen condition.

Liver Meridian

The main function of the Liver is to store and filter the blood. The Liver is one of the main storage places for blood, and helps control the amount of blood according to the activity of the human body. A person whose Liver is balanced has strong psychological constitution and psychological resilience. The Liver is closely associated with anger. The Liver also has a very close connection to muscle, nail and eye condition. Liver irregularity often shows in the nails of the hands and feet. Blurred vision, dizziness, extremely dry eyes and low night vision also point to a Liver imbalance.

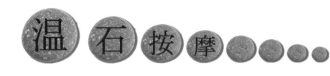

21

Lesson Twenty-One

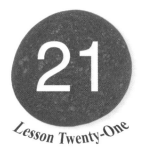

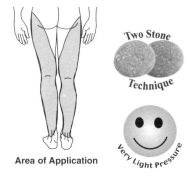

Area of Application

Two Stone Technique

Very Light Pressure

温石軽擦法
Light Stroking Over the Posterior Leg

Begin Japanese Hot Stone Massage on the posterior leg by applying light, smooth, long strokes over the entire calf and thigh region. This stroke evenly disperses the temperature of the stones. The next techniques are kneading and pressure techniques, which require the stones to stay in one place for a long period of time. Therefore, the stones must cool enough that your client doesn't experience discomfort. Use caution while working the medial thigh, due to its hypersensitivity to high temperatures, and to respect the modesty of your client. The medial thigh, like other areas with limited exposure, can be very sensitive to touch and temperature changes. Unless specific work is required, you should limit work in this area. We recommend following the posterior center of the thigh along the Bladder meridian with one stone. Simultaneously stroke the lateral side of the thigh over the Gall Bladder meridian at the iliotibial tract with the other stone. Twisting your wrist while switching directions during this stroke will create unnecessary tension. A correct body position is crucial for smoothly completing this stroke. Keep your stance wide enough to smoothly accommodate your movements from the beginning to the end of the stroke. Refrain from bending over during this stroke to minimize stress on your back. All upper body and arm movements are initiated from the legs and hips.

Step 1

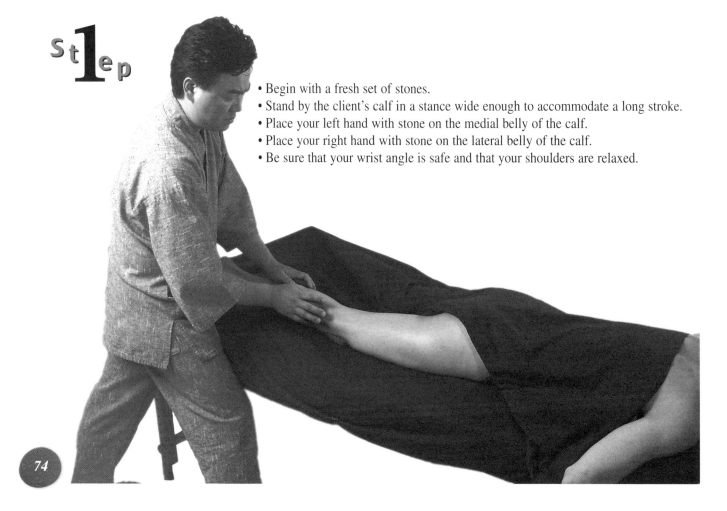

- Begin with a fresh set of stones.
- Stand by the client's calf in a stance wide enough to accommodate a long stroke.
- Place your left hand with stone on the medial belly of the calf.
- Place your right hand with stone on the lateral belly of the calf.
- Be sure that your wrist angle is safe and that your shoulders are relaxed.

Step 2
- Simultaneously stroke both hands in a superior direction toward the hip.
- Keep your wrists flexible, so your hands can contour the client's legs.
- Lighten your stroke over bony surfaces.

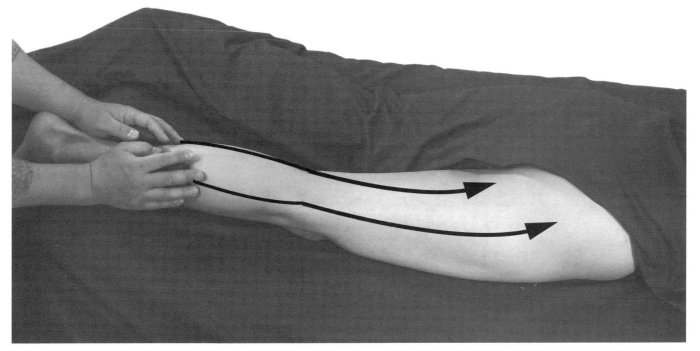

Step 3
- At the glutes, reverse the direction and stroke inferiorly.
- Reduce your pressure on the return stroke.
- Repeat and reposition your hands to cover the entire area.
- Continue until the stone temperature is correct for the next technique.

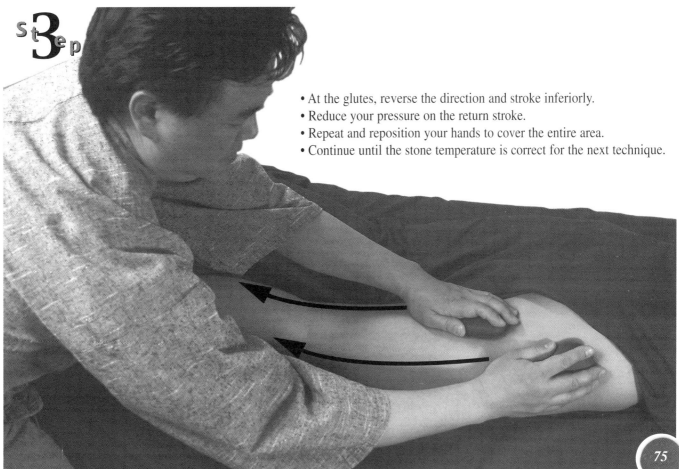

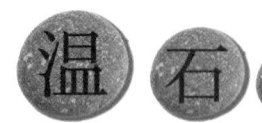

22

Lesson Twenty-Two

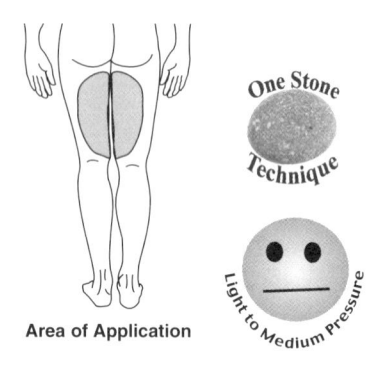

Area of Application

One Stone Technique

Light to Medium Pressure

温石揉提法
Rotation Over the Medial Hamstrings

Apply this technique from across the massage table using only one stone. Applying the technique in this manner allows you to stand directly in front of the leg on which you are working. This position prevents wrist distortions and allows you to provide a full range of pressure. Lowering your body position and keeping your shoulders dropped also ensures proper wrist alignment. During this lesson, the stones do not slide over the skin; instead, they engage the underlying tissue, at which point the rotation is initiated. The medial hamstring is a hypersensitive zone; therefore, use caution when applying high temperatures or pressure to this region. In areas where draping and high temperatures are concerns, you may perform this technique over the sheets. The diameter of rotation for this technique is determined by the size and tone of your client's thighs. For some clients, you must sink through the adipose to engage the underlying muscle structure. In this instance, decrease rotation diameter accordingly and take the same precautions in areas with excessive body hair. Begin with relatively light pressure, then gradually increase pressure as the tissue relaxes.

Step 1

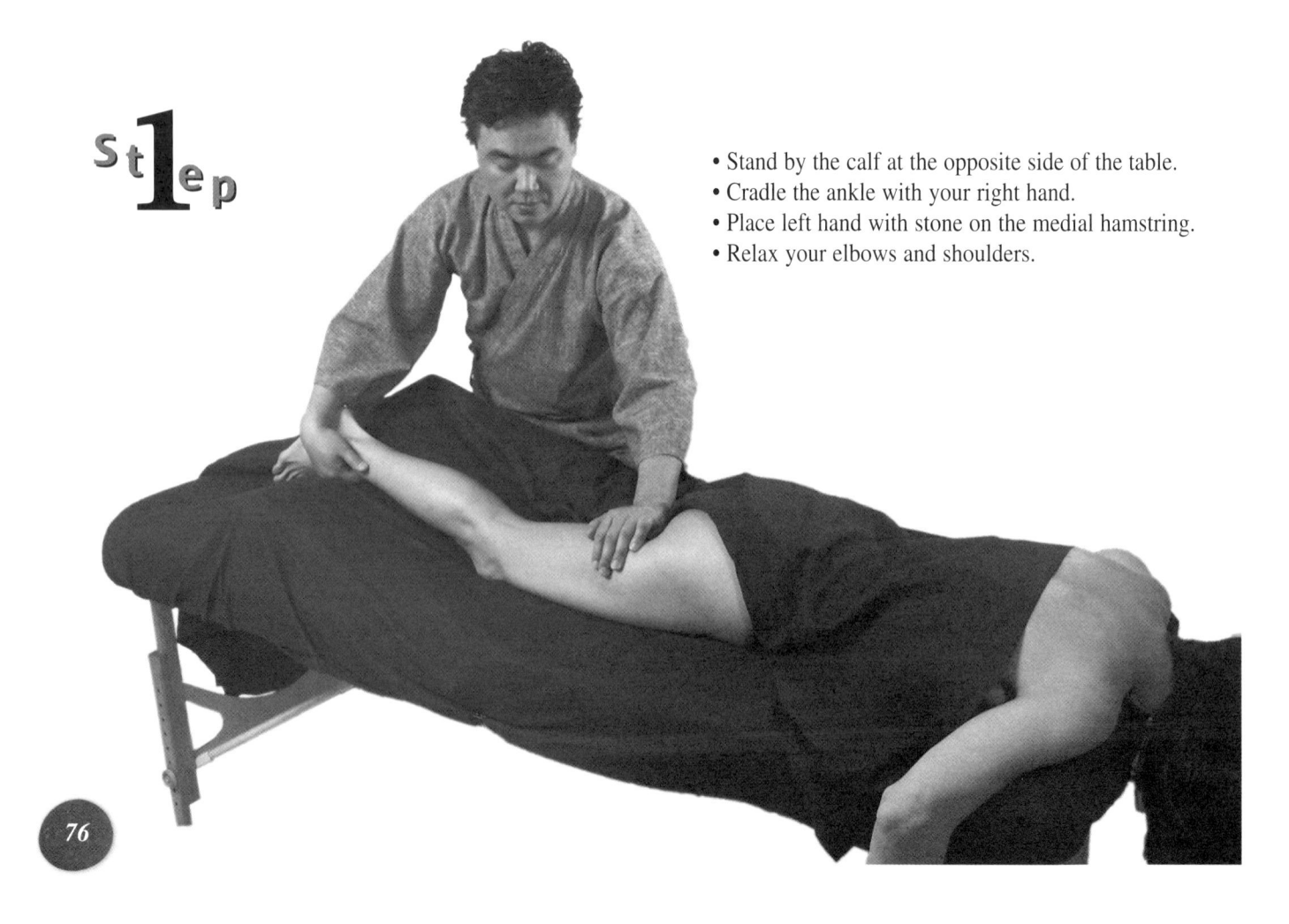

- Stand by the calf at the opposite side of the table.
- Cradle the ankle with your right hand.
- Place left hand with stone on the medial hamstring.
- Relax your elbows and shoulders.

Step 2

- Apply pressure to engage the underlying tissue.
- Rotate in a superior, then lateral direction.
- Do not hyperabduct your wrist.

Step 3

- Continue rotating inferiorly, then medially.
- Repeat five to seven times.
- Relax your wrist and shoulder.

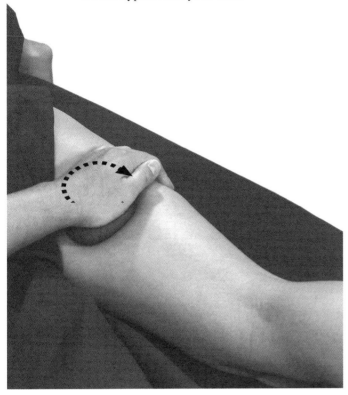

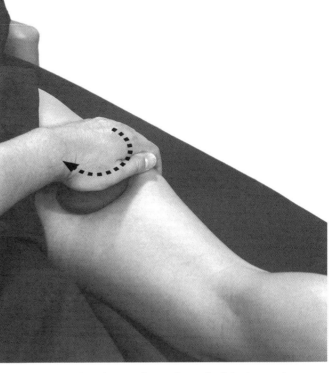

Step 4

- Reposition one hand-width inferior.
- Repeat rotation.

Step 5

- Continue series to the end of the hamstrings.
- Do not apply pressure to the posterior knee.

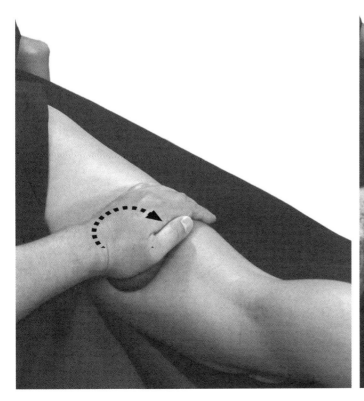

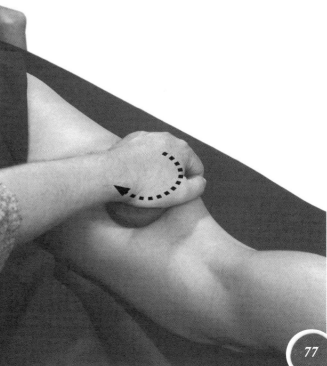

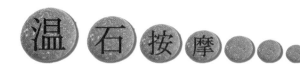

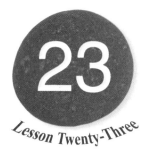

Lesson Twenty-Three

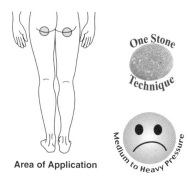

Area of Application

One Stone Technique

Medium to Heavy Pressure

温石圧迫法
Pressure on *Sho Fu* (Bladder-36)

This technique is often used in combination with the previous lesson. The *sho fu* tsubo point is located at the midline of the upper leg on the ischial tuberosity of the Bladder meridian. This tsubo belongs to the Bladder meridian, and is traditionally used to release low back and psoas tension. Applying pressure at *sho fu* is an effective alternative to direct low back techniques, which may be too invasive when low back injuries are acute. Releasing the hips using *sho fu* will allow the low back to relax, thereby facilitating further work. As you master this technique, you will learn to perform smooth, rocking rotations at *sho fu,* while simultaneously rotating the ankle to increase effectiveness. Gentle rocking will also minimize any sensitivity your client may feel when pressure is applied to this tsubo point. Achieve proper wrist alignment by keeping your arm in a parallel orientation to the leg. Holding your arm perpendicular to the leg forces your elbow up and causes wrist hyperextension.

承扶
Sho Fu
Bladder-36

Sho Fu is located on the crease between the hips and legs, midway between the lateral edge of the hip. This point is located on the ischial tuberosity.

S t **1** e p

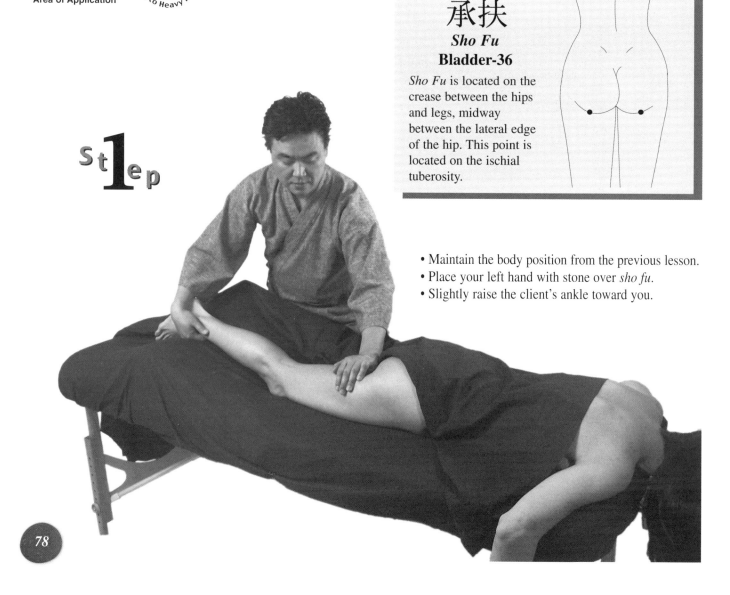

• Maintain the body position from the previous lesson.
• Place your left hand with stone over *sho fu*.
• Slightly raise the client's ankle toward you.

温石按摩

Step 2

- Apply pressure with your left hand in a supra-lateral direction.
- Rotate the client's heel toward you, while adding slight traction.

Step 3

- Hold the stretch for a few seconds, then release.
- Repeat two to three times.

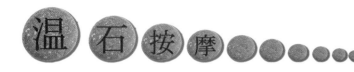

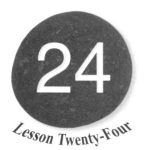

温石揉提法
Rotation Over the Lateral Thigh and Gluteals

After the medial thigh muscles are sufficiently warmed from across the body, return to the side of the table with the exposed leg. This is a one-hand rotation technique in which your lateral hand applies rotation, while the opposite hand supports and stabilizes the leg. Stabilizing the leg minimizes leg movement and prevents excessive wrist strain during rotation. A warm stone in your stabilizing hand can further facilitate a hamstring release.

Prevent wrist hyperextension when accommodating larger clients, by dropping your stance and sinking into the tissue, before beginning rotation. Lowering your stance and keeping your elbows dropped and relaxed will also ensure modest finger placement at the client's medial glutes. Rotation is achieved by using larger hip and shoulder muscles and should not come from your wrists. Broad rotations may be performed with light pressure, and as pressure increases, rotation diameter decreases. When applying deep pressure, keep your wrists straight and flat, as to not block *ki* flow.

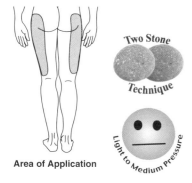

Area of Application

Two Stone Technique

Light to Medium Pressure

Step 1

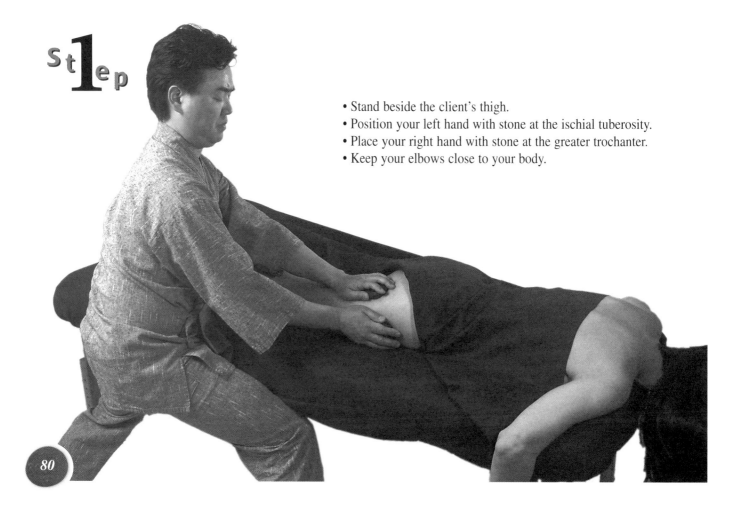

- Stand beside the client's thigh.
- Position your left hand with stone at the ischial tuberosity.
- Place your right hand with stone at the greater trochanter.
- Keep your elbows close to your body.

温石按摩

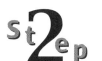

- Apply pressure with your right hand to engage the underlying tissue.
- Rotate in a superior, then medial direction.
- Anchor your fingers to localize your palm rotation.

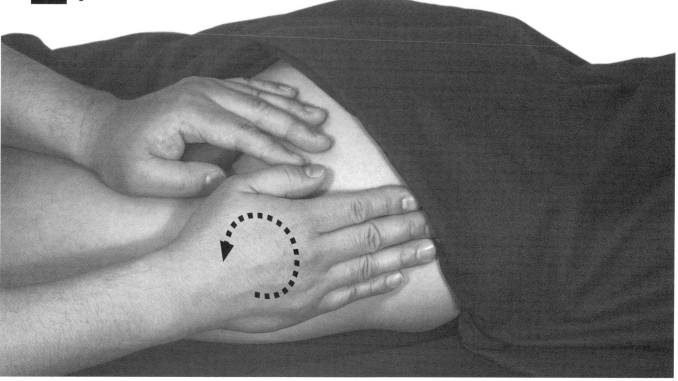

- Complete the rotation by moving inferiorly, then laterally; repeat eight to ten rotations.
- Continue rotating as you gradually reposition your hands inferiorly along the lateral thigh.

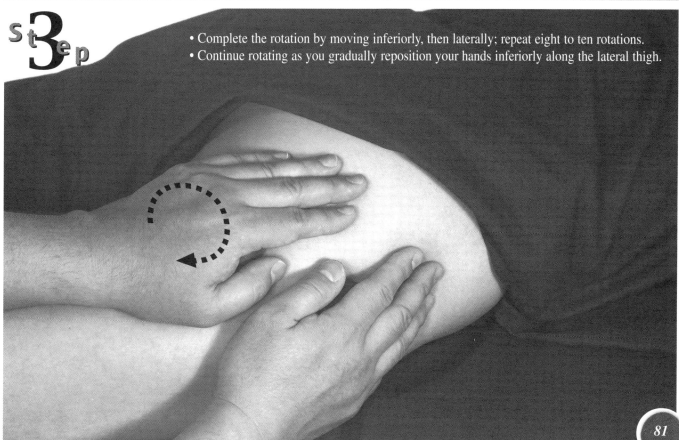

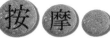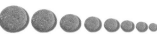

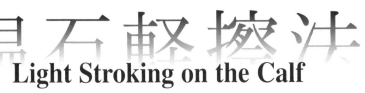

Light Stroking on the Calf

25

Lesson Twenty-Five

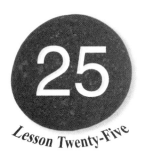

Area of Application

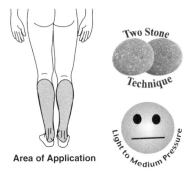

Two Stone Technique

Light to Medium Pressure

Because we are beginning work on a new region of the body, you should begin this technique with fresh hot stones. Place the stones on both sides of the calf to contact three seperate meridians. The lateral stroke follows the Bladder meridian, while the medial stroke moves along either the Kidney meridian or the Spleen meridian. Continue stroking until your new stones have cooled to a temperature that is appropriate for deeper techniques. The speed of your stroke should once again correspond to the temperature of the stones. Stroke lightly and/or more quickly with hot stones, and gradually slow down and/or increase pressure as the stones cool. The medial calf is extremely sensitive for some individuals, so adjust your pressure accordingly. Avoid contacting the malleoli of the lower leg, the patella and any other bony surfaces with the stones, because this can be very uncomfortable. Your arms should not supply the primary strength for this stroke; instead, move your entire body to create a smooth, continuous movement.

Step 1

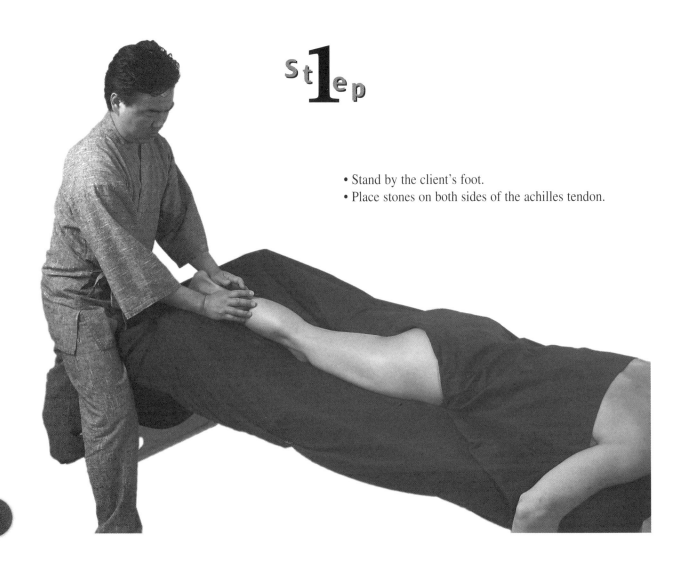

• Stand by the client's foot.
• Place stones on both sides of the achilles tendon.

温石按摩

Step 2

• Stroke superiorly on both sides of the calf.
• Relax your elbows and wrists, so your hands can contour the leg.

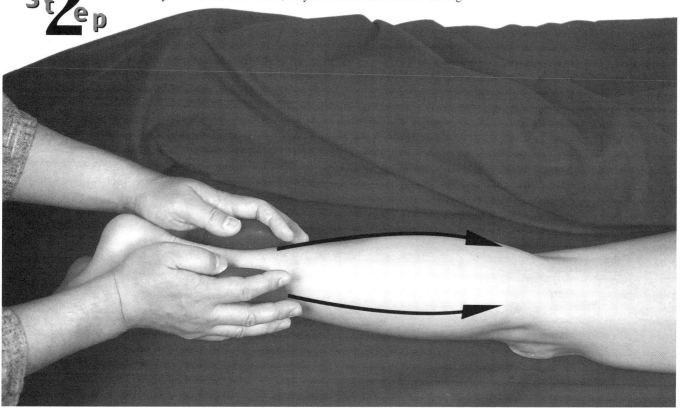

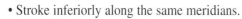

Step 3

• Stroke inferiorly along the same meridians.
• Repeat the stroke eight to ten times to address both medial meridians.

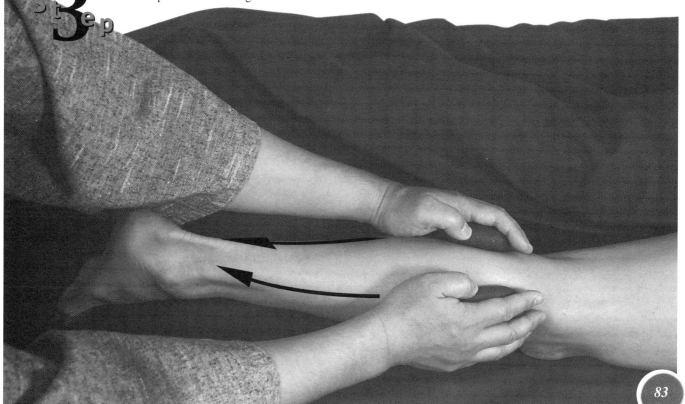

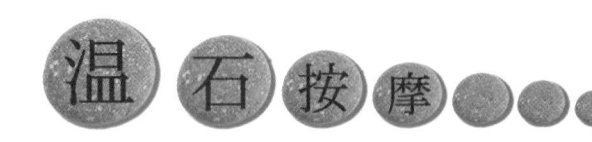

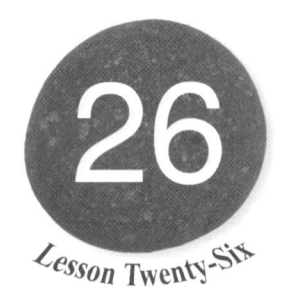

Lesson Twenty-Six

温石揉提法
Rotation on the Sides of the Calf

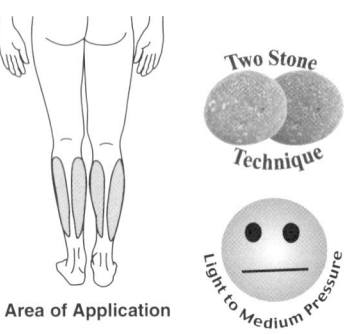

Area of Application

Two Stone Technique

Light to Medium Pressure

The calf muscle, which is composed of the gastrocnemius and soleus, can be the source of many problems. Long hours of standing or exercise often create calf tension. The calves are especially problematic when the arches of the feet are stressed. Conditions, such as flat feet or pelvic misalignment, can also result in tight calves. Chronic and excessive calf tension may also indicate lower extremity misalignment. It is important to note, however, that high levels of tension can also be caused by exercise, such as running, and do not necessarily reflect poor structural alignment. To effectively release the calves, apply this technique intermittently, and in combination with the next two examples. Releasing tension from the feet, pelvis and lower back will also facilitate the release of calf tension. The medial calf, and the soleus in particular, are often very sensitive, so check your pressure and evaluate your client's non-verbal responses accordingly. This technique requires more movement and longer strokes, so avoid contacting bony structures with stones.

Step 1

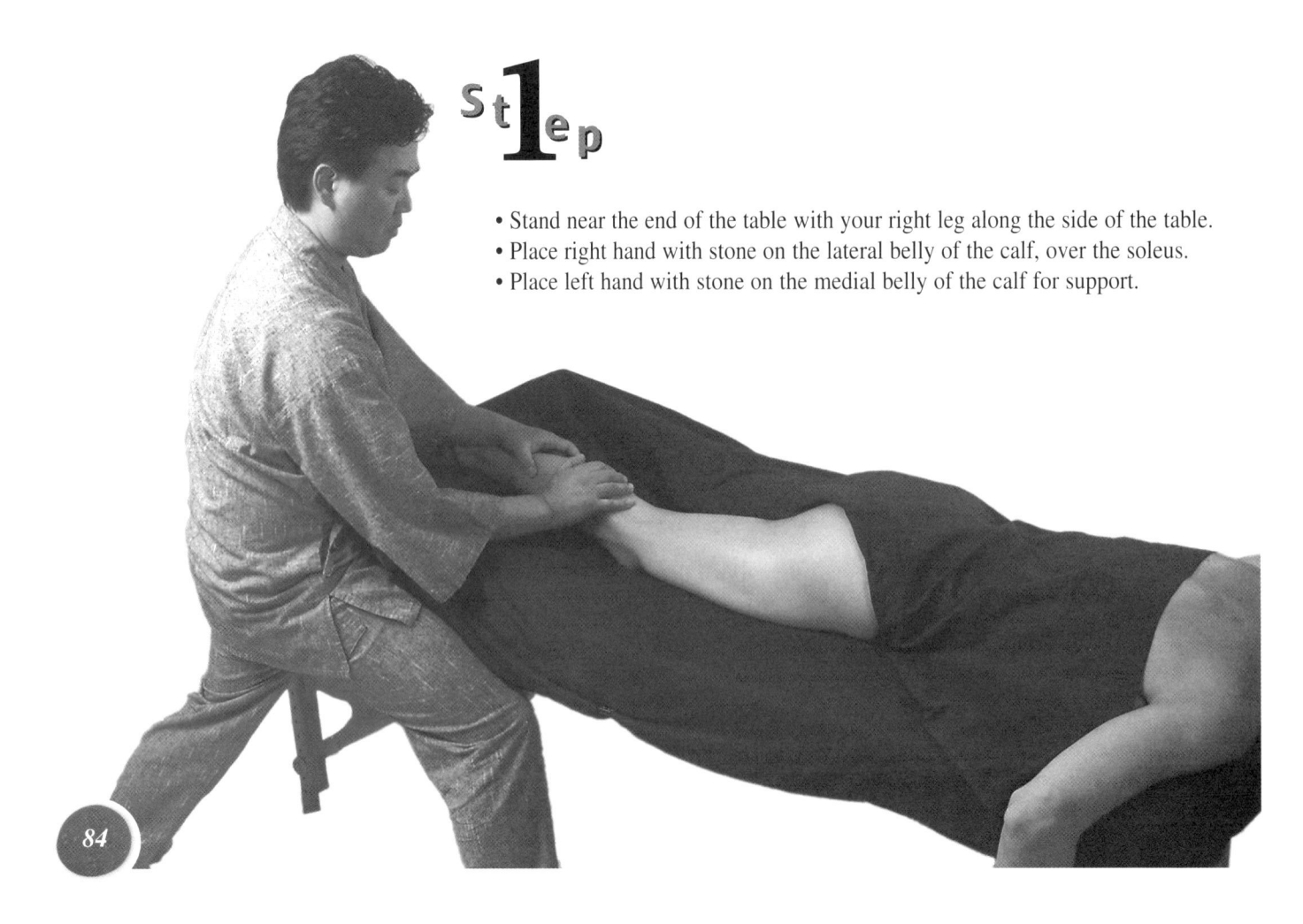

- Stand near the end of the table with your right leg along the side of the table.
- Place right hand with stone on the lateral belly of the calf, over the soleus.
- Place left hand with stone on the medial belly of the calf for support.

Step 2
- Apply pressure with your right hand to engage the underlying tissue.
- From the side, rotate superiorly and posteriorly.
- Keep your hands aligned with the arms.

Step 3
- Complete the rotation inferiorly and anteriorly.
- Repeat the rotation three to five times.
- Reposition stones inferiorly and repeat.
- Do not contact the fibula with the stones.

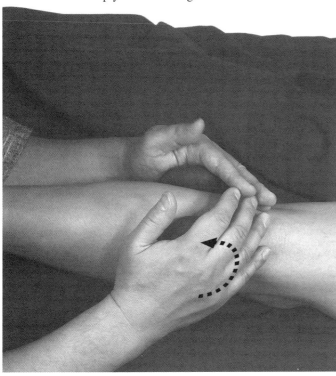

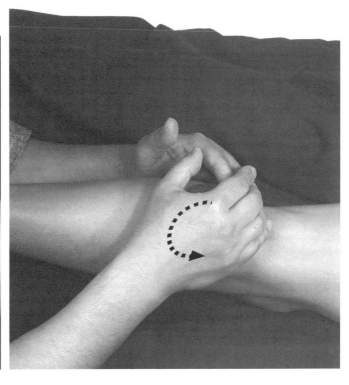

Step 4
- Rotate on the medial calf with your left hand.
- Rotate superiorly, then posteriorly.

Step 5
- Complete the rotation inferiorly and anteriorly.
- Reposition inferiorly and repeat.

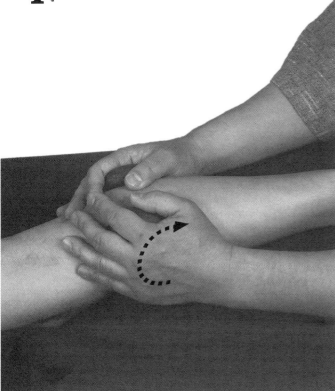

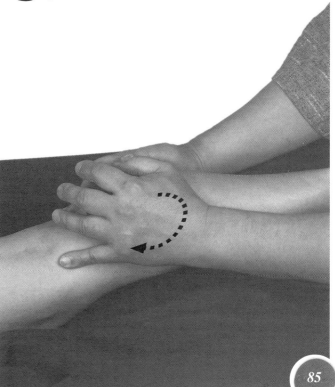

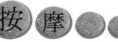

温石揉提法
Rotation on the Center of the Calf

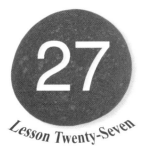

27
Lesson Twenty-Seven

Combine this technique with the previous lesson to release muscular tension in the gastrocnemius and soleus. This technique may be performed with the leg resting on the bolster; however, take care not to hyperextend your wrist. Maintain wrist alignment by adjusting your stance and the angle of your body. This technique follows the Bladder meridian at the center of the calf.

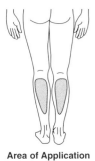

Area of Application

One Stone Technique

Light to Medium Pressure

In traditional Japanese massage, therapists also elevate the client's calf. Elevating allows the therapist to pull and engage the underlying tissues, while the client's leg remains relaxed.

Step 1

- Stand at the end of the table, beside the client's calf.
- Place your right hand with stone on the calf.
- Place your left hand next to the stone for support.

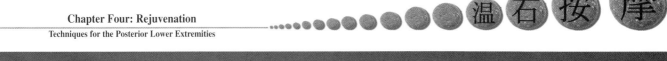

温石按摩

Step 2

- Apply pressure with your right hand to engage the underlying tissue.
- Begin small, circular rotations and repeat five to seven times.

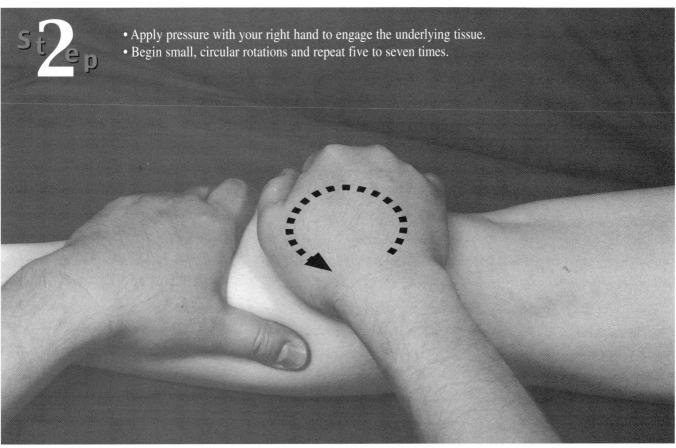

Step 3

- Reposition one stone-width inferior and repeat.
- Continue until you reach the achilles tendon.
- Repeat the entire procedure three to five times.

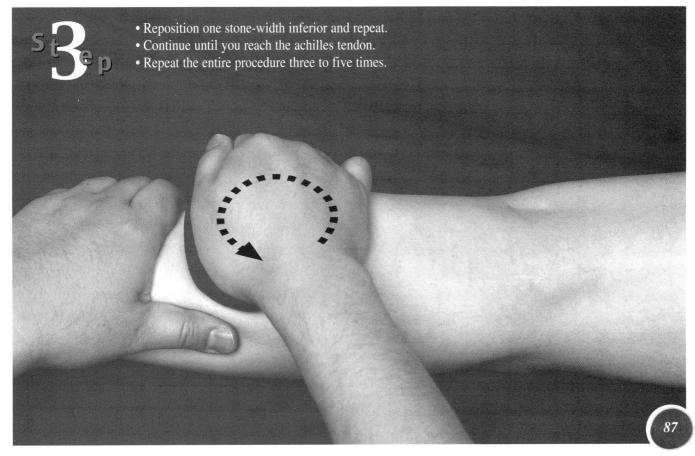

87

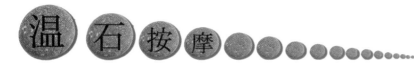

28

Lesson Twenty-Eight

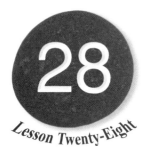

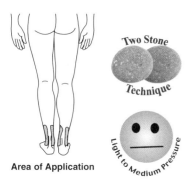

Area of Application

Two Stone Technique

Light to Medium Pressure

Compress and Vibrate the Achilles Tendon

Among the many methods of manipulating the achilles tendon, compression and vibration are some of the simplest, yet most effective techniques. Vibration is extremely helpful for stagnant *ki* flow and is used frequently during Japanese massage. Vibration allows you to deeply penetrate, while reducing pressure. Vibration releases muscle tissue by bombarding the nervous system with signals, which causes fatigue. When the nerves fatigue, muscle tension releases. Vibration is created by contracting core and extremity muscles, resulting in a subtle vibration, which is directed onto client during treatment. Vibration techniques are optional, because they can be difficult to learn and take practice to apply effectively. Compression with hot stones is another subtle, yet effective method for contacting deeper muscle tissue. In this case, compression is performed simply from the weight of your hands and the hot stones over the achilles. To avoid unsafe wrist angles, lower your stance, drop your shoulders and keep your elbows close to your sides.

Step 1

- Stand at the foot of the table.
- Place palms with stones around the achilles tendon and interlace your fingers.

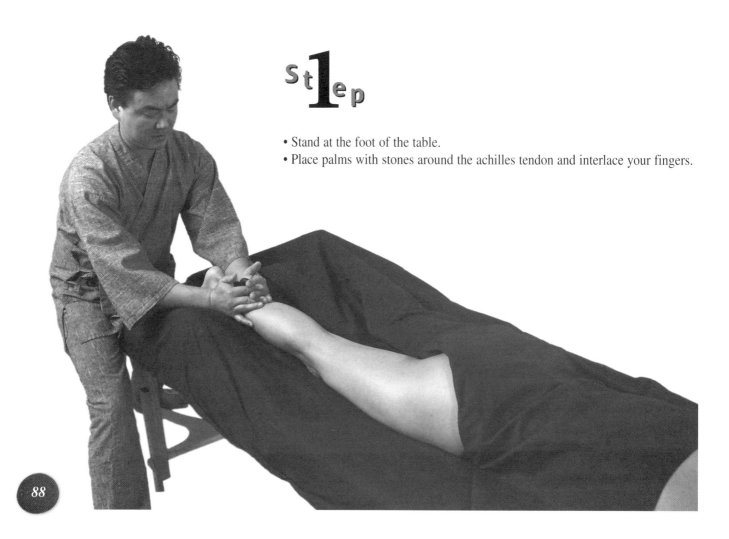

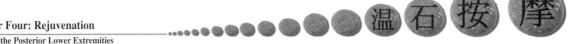

温石按摩

Step 2

- Apply equal pressure to both sides of the tendon simultaneously.
- Maintain pressure for three to five seconds.
- Apply vibration near the end of the compression, then release.
- Reposition one stone-width inferior and repeat.

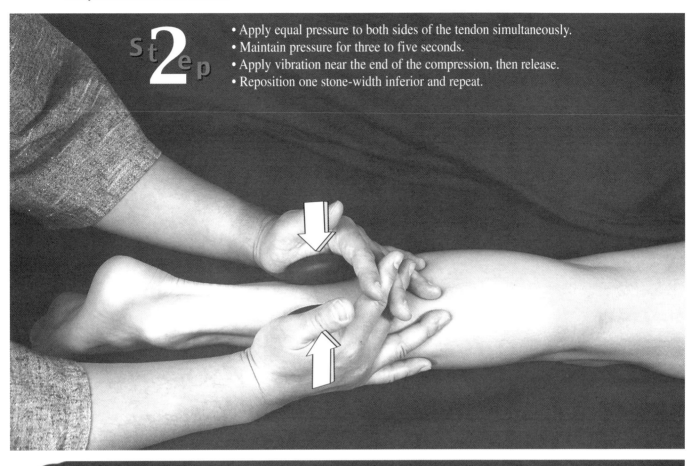

Step 3

- Reposition about one stone-width inferior and repeat the compression.
- Continue repositioning and apply compression to cover the entire length of the tendon.
- Avoid contacting the malleoli with the stones.

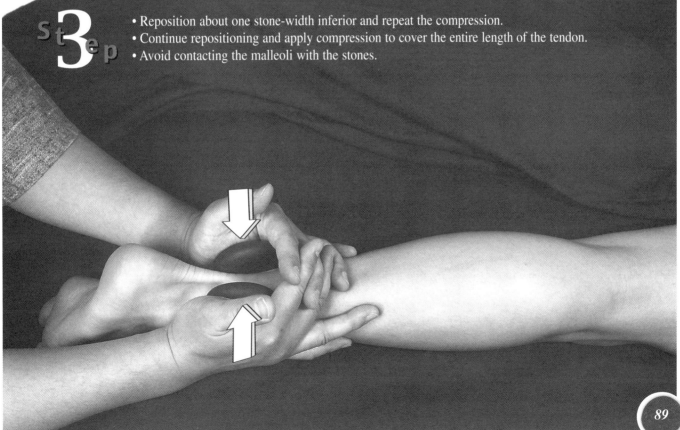

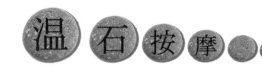
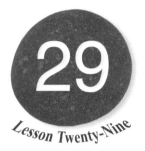

29

Lesson Twenty-Nine

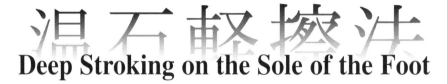

Deep Stroking on the Sole of the Foot

Use fresh hot stones when applying this technique and begin quick, superficial strokes over the entire sole of the foot. Only proceed as outlined in the following steps when your stone has cooled to an appropriate temperature. Traditional Japanese massage uses meridians and tsubo in the feet and ankles to treat numerous health conditions. Foot massage is one of the simplest, yet most effective methods for increasing overall health. Always note the condition of your client's feet; if the if the condition is questionable, apply these techniques through a sheet or other protective barrier.

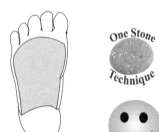

Area of Application

One Stone Technique

Very Light Pressure

Step 1

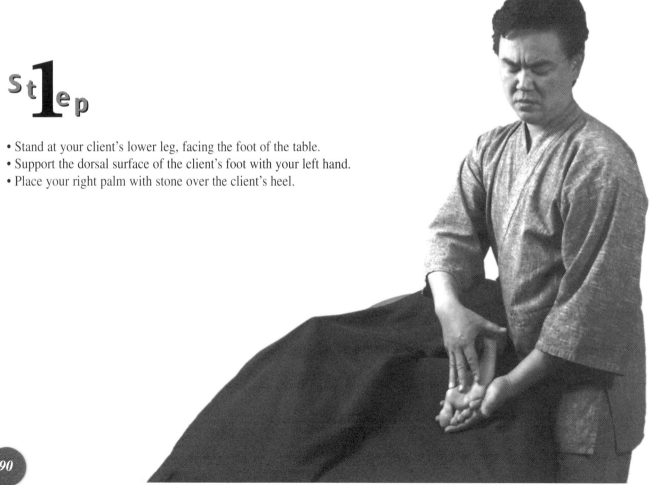

- Stand at your client's lower leg, facing the foot of the table.
- Support the dorsal surface of the client's foot with your left hand.
- Place your right palm with stone over the client's heel.

温石按摩

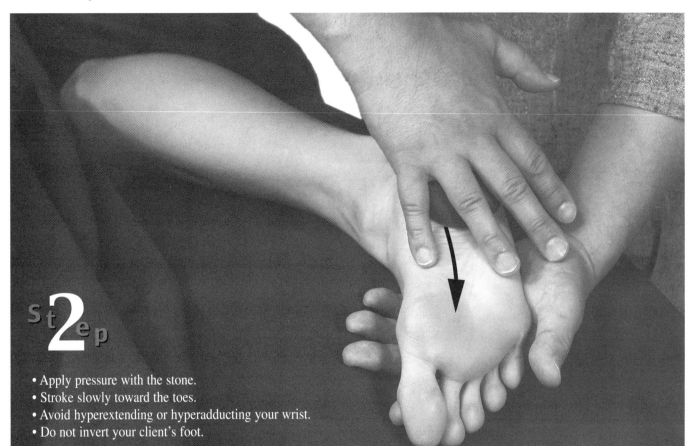

Step 2

- Apply pressure with the stone.
- Stroke slowly toward the toes.
- Avoid hyperextending or hyperadducting your wrist.
- Do not invert your client's foot.

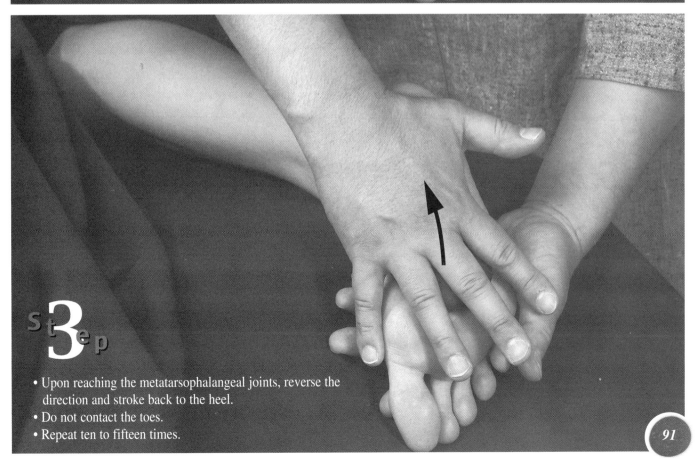

Step 3

- Upon reaching the metatarsophalangeal joints, reverse the direction and stroke back to the heel.
- Do not contact the toes.
- Repeat ten to fifteen times.

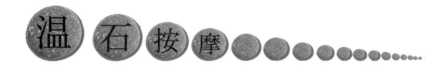

温石揉提法
Deep Rotation on the Arch with One Stone

Lesson Thirty

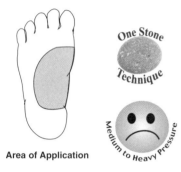

Area of Application

One Stone Technique

Medium to Heavy Pressure

The feet are the foundation of the human structure. They support the entire skeleton and are crucial for maintaining proper knee, hip and body alignment. This technique is used in combination with other techniques to reduce muscle tension, increase joint mobility and restore balance and body alignment. You can apply many Japanese massage techniques to the feet with hot stones. Hot stone foot massage is also a wonderful addition to any pedicure or facial treatment. You can also greatly enhance your hot stone foot massage treatment, by incorporating hot stone shiatsu into your practice. *Shiatsu for the Feet* is an easy to follow, step-by-step guide that introduces tsubo point locations and treatment techniques. You can apply this technique very deeply; however, you must keep your pressure within your client's tolerance level and a therapeutic range. If your hand becomes fatigued during this application, alternate hands or reposition the stone in your hand. When applied within therapeutic levels, this technique can be very effective for plantar fascitis; however, you must be very sensitive to your client's condition.

Step 1

• Maintain the body position from the previous lesson.
• Use your fingers to secure the stone in the palm of your right hand.
• Extend a small portion of the stone beyond the bottom of your hand.
• Place the stone on the proximal edge of the arch, near the heel.

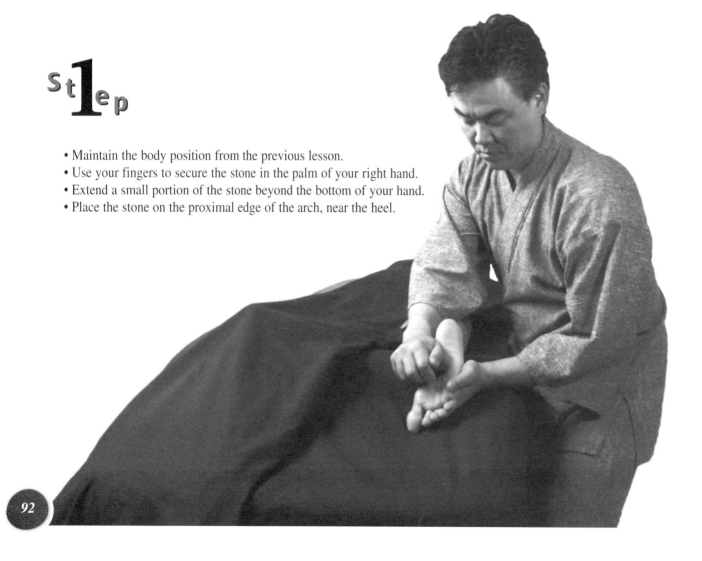

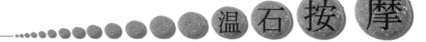

温石按摩

Step 2

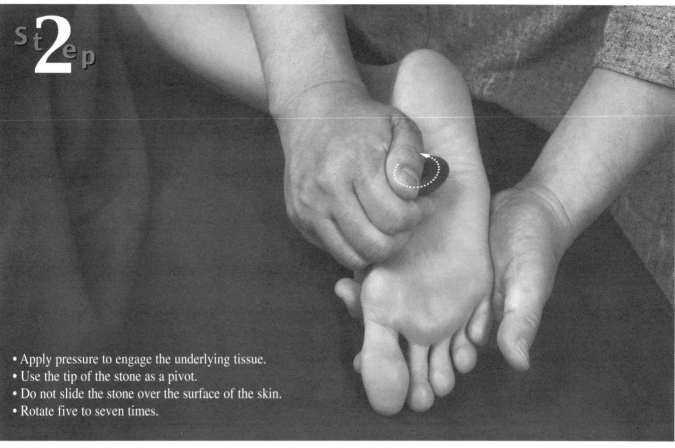

- Apply pressure to engage the underlying tissue.
- Use the tip of the stone as a pivot.
- Do not slide the stone over the surface of the skin.
- Rotate five to seven times.

Step 3

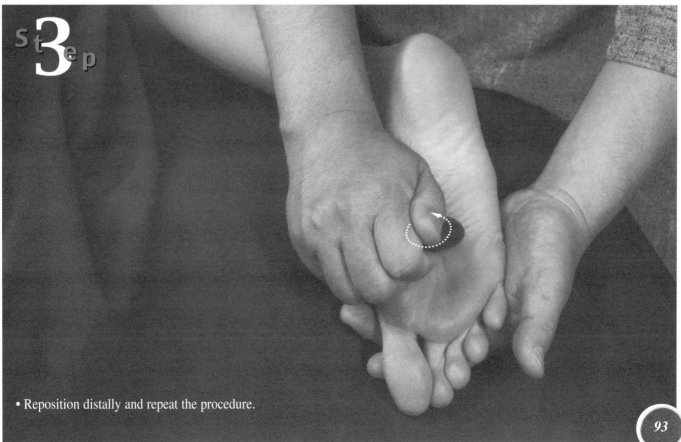

- Reposition distally and repeat the procedure.

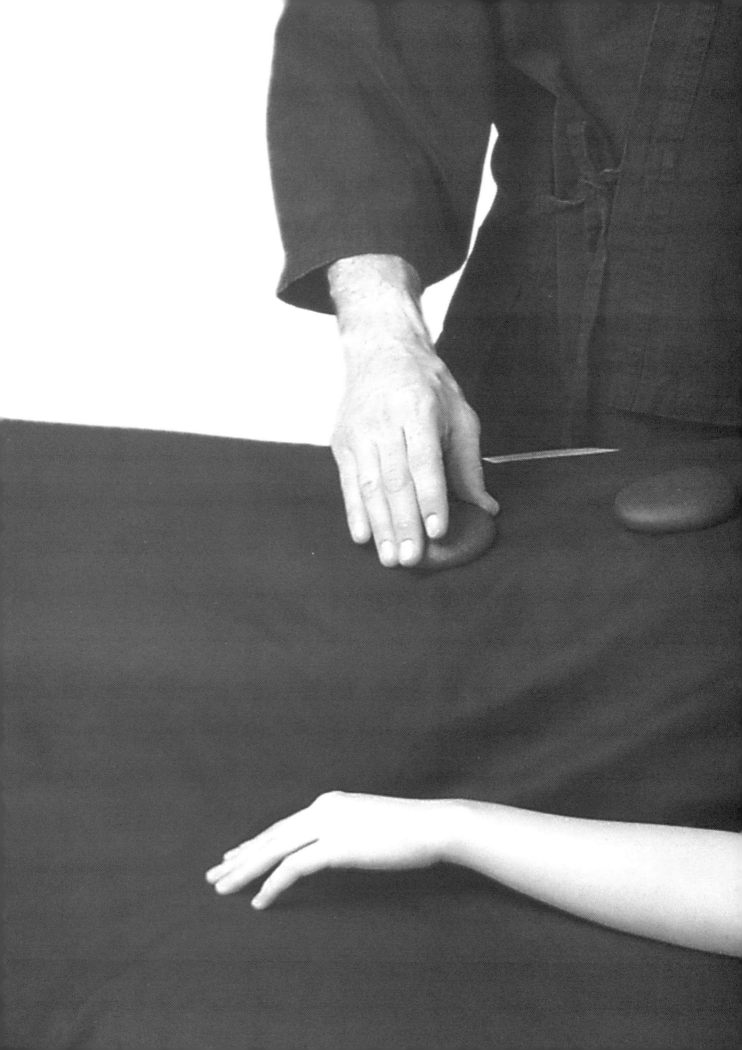

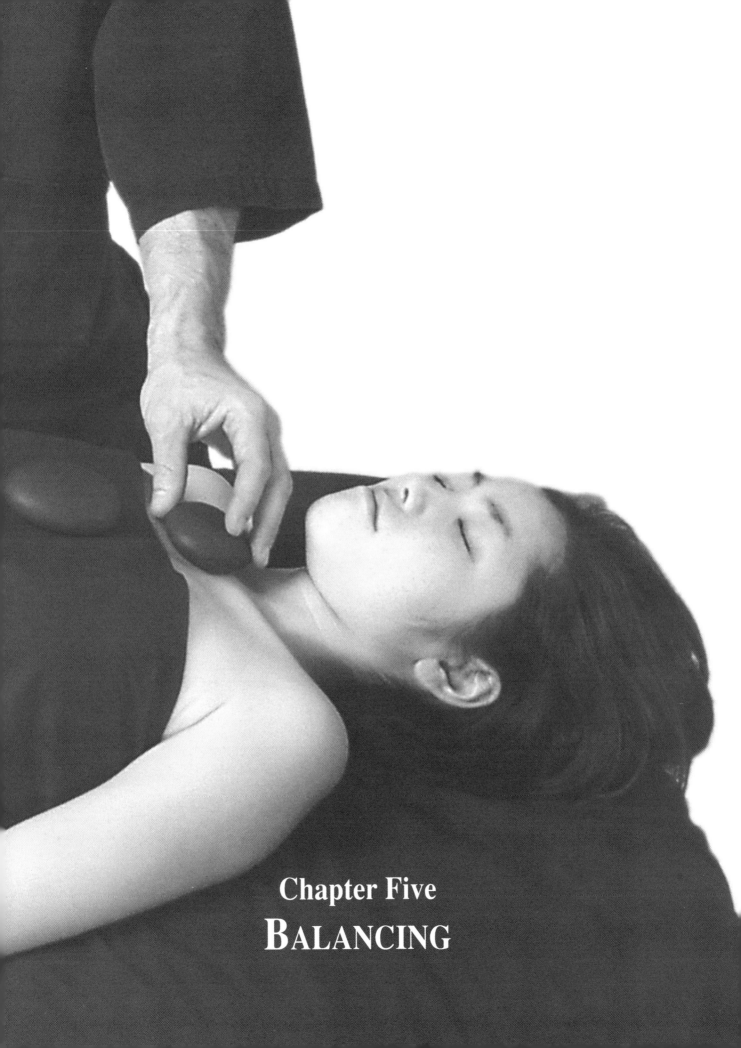

Chapter Five
BALANCING

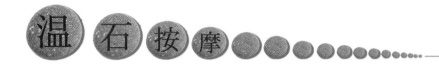

Chapter Five

BALANCING

Techniques for the Anterior Upper Extremities

In this chapter, we introduce ten techniques for the upper anterior torso. Metal, one of the five elements, represents harmony between the elements and balance between *yin* and *yang*. Asian medicine is not concerned with good, bad, better or worse, because everything is about balance. Excessive conditions are as much of a problem as depleted conditions. As we explained for *yin/yang* theory, it is important to achieve harmony between *yin* and *yang* within one treatment. This chapter deals with the *yin* portion of treatment, which includes subtle, gentle, calming techniques. This Japanese Hot Stone Massage treatment began with stronger *yang* techniques in the Passion Chapter, and now moves toward gentle, balancing *yin* techniques.

The first seven techniques balance meridians in the arms. There are three *yin* meridians and three *yang* meridians in the arms, but only the three *yin* meridians maintain proper balance and healthy condition.

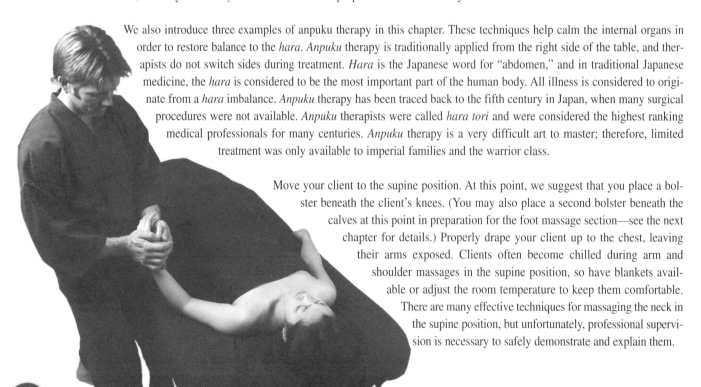

We also introduce three examples of anpuku therapy in this chapter. These techniques help calm the internal organs in order to restore balance to the *hara*. *Anpuku* therapy is traditionally applied from the right side of the table, and therapists do not switch sides during treatment. *Hara* is the Japanese word for "abdomen," and in traditional Japanese medicine, the *hara* is considered to be the most important part of the human body. All illness is considered to originate from a *hara* imbalance. *Anpuku* therapy has been traced back to the fifth century in Japan, when many surgical procedures were not available. *Anpuku* therapists were called *hara tori* and were considered the highest ranking medical professionals for many centuries. *Anpuku* therapy is a very difficult art to master; therefore, limited treatment was only available to imperial families and the warrior class.

Move your client to the supine position. At this point, we suggest that you place a bolster beneath the client's knees. (You may also place a second bolster beneath the calves at this point in preparation for the foot massage section—see the next chapter for details.) Properly drape your client up to the chest, leaving their arms exposed. Clients often become chilled during arm and shoulder massages in the supine position, so have blankets available or adjust the room temperature to keep them comfortable. There are many effective techniques for massaging the neck in the supine position, but unfortunately, professional supervision is necessary to safely demonstrate and explain them.

温 石 按 摩

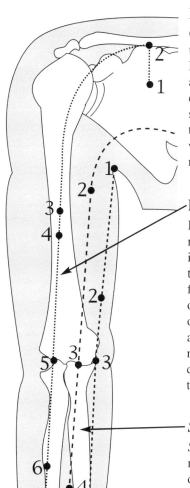

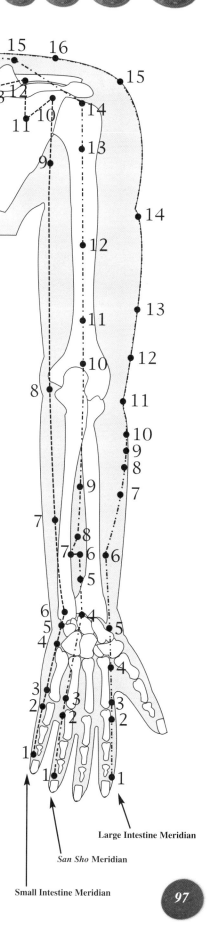

Meridians in the Arms

Of the six meridians that run through the arms, the three *yang* meridians— Large Intestine, *San Sho* (Triple Heater) and Small Intestine—are previously explained in Chapter Three. In the supine position, we primarily deal with the three *yin* meridians in the arms, which are the Lung, *Shin Po* and Heart meridians.

Lung Meridian

In Asian medicine, the Lung meridian represents the entire respiratory system, including the nose, nasal passages, throat, bronchial passage and the surface of the skin. The Lung is in charge of taking in air *ki*, which is very close to oxygen, and eliminating carbon dioxide and heat. The Lung is also closely connected with sadness. Excess sadness or depression can be helped or treated with this meridian.

Shin Po Meridian

Shin Po, like *San Sho*, does not have a material equivalent in Western physiology. *Shin Po* is often mistranslated as "Pericardium meridian," "Heart Protector," "Heart Constrictor" or even "Circulation-Sex," even though this meridian has nothing to do with circulation or sex. The main function of *Shin Po* is to protect and support heart function, because the heart can not withstand significant stress.

Heart Meridian

The Heart, in Asian Medicine, is the master of all internal organs. As the main energy chamber for all *ki* energy, the Heart produces primary functioning *ki* for the human body. By collecting heaven *ki* (air *ki*) from the Lungs and earth *ki* (food essence) from the Small Intestine, the Heart creates the primary energy used for all human functions. The Heart governs Blood pulsations and controls the speed and amount of Blood that circulates throughout the body. The Heart also stores *Shin*, which is the center of your spirituality.

Large Intestine Meridian

San Sho Meridian

Small Intestine Meridian

97

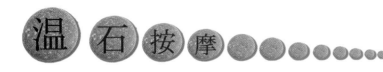

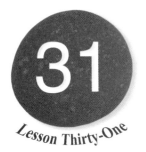

(31)

Lesson Thirty-One

温石軽擦法
Light Stroking Over the Arm and Shoulder

Apply this light, stroking technique over the entire arm with a fresh set of stones. When possible, this stroke contours the entire region, from the wrist to the rotator cuff. Adjust your client's arm to maximize surface area and increase effectiveness. To create a smooth movement, do not hunch over while stroking. Maintain a relatively wide stance, lower your pelvis and move your body forward as you stroke. Bring your body back toward you at the end of the stroke to prevent wrist hyperextension. Initiate this stroke with your entire body movement, not just hand and arm movement. If you are small or short, or if you are massaging an extremely large client, divide the stroke into two parts, as necessary. When contouring the arm, stroke lightly around bony landmarks, especially the shoulder and wrist regions. Maintain proper wrist alignment to avoid hyperadduction or hyperabduction.

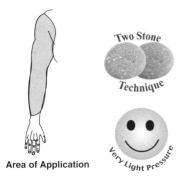

Area of Application

Two Stone Technique

Very Light Pressure

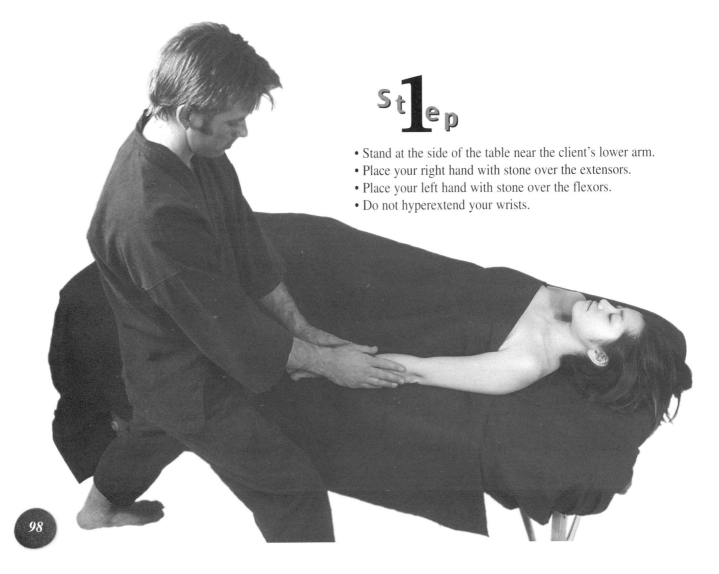

St**1**ep

- Stand at the side of the table near the client's lower arm.
- Place your right hand with stone over the extensors.
- Place your left hand with stone over the flexors.
- Do not hyperextend your wrists.

温石按摩

• Stroke from the wrist to the shoulder with both hands simultaneously.
• Keep your wrists flexible to accommodate the contours of the arm.

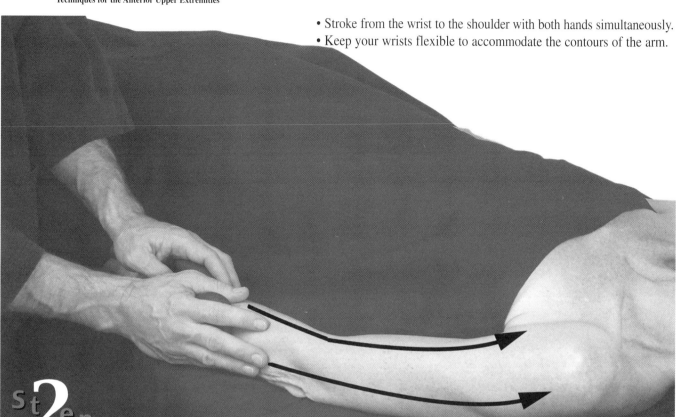

Step 2

• When you reach the deltoid region, reverse and stroke toward the wrist.
• Repeat until the stones are a comfortable temperature for the next technique.
  • As you repeat, slightly adjust your path to accommodate different aspects of the arm.

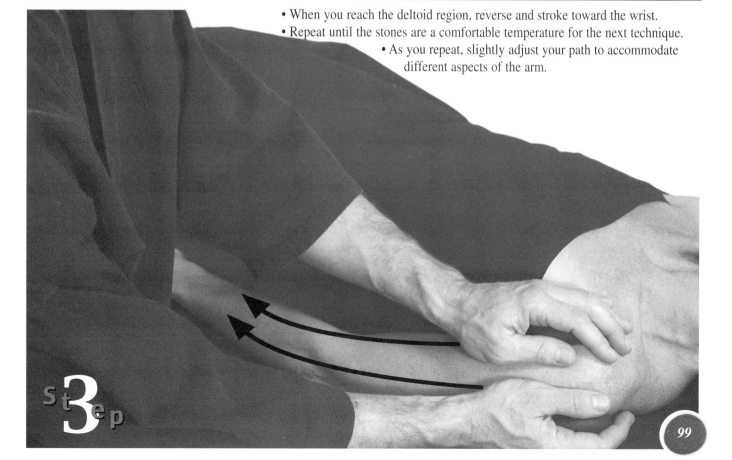

Step 3

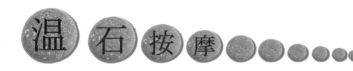

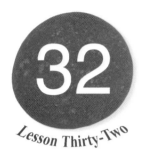

32

Lesson Thirty-Two

温石圧迫法
Kenbiki Technique on the Pectoralis

Kenbiki is a unique Japanese massage technique that combines kneading, pressure or vibration with rotation and gentle traction. This is a difficult technique to master, and achieving pressure and traction synchroneity requires significant practice. This technique effectively loosens the pectoralis muscle, while restoring shoulder mobility with minimal discomfort. Many people are sensitive in this area, so proceed slowly and gently. Begin with light pressure and small movements, then as your client relaxes, increase the pressure and range of motion. If your client has large breasts, tuck the drape under the scapula or ask them to hold the tissue in an inferior-medial direction to prevent treatment interferences. Reverse your leg position to create proper traction for this technique. Stand near the lower rib cage with your left hand and stone over the pectoral region.

Area of Application

One Stone Technique

Light to Medium Pressure

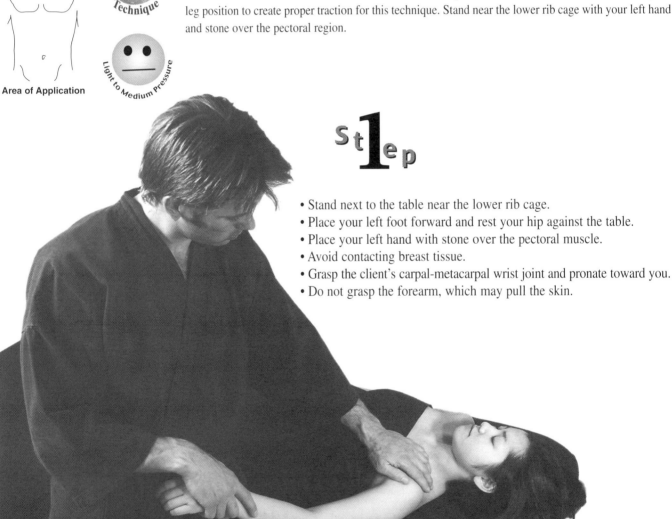

St**1**ep

- Stand next to the table near the lower rib cage.
- Place your left foot forward and rest your hip against the table.
- Place your left hand with stone over the pectoral muscle.
- Avoid contacting breast tissue.
- Grasp the client's carpal-metacarpal wrist joint and pronate toward you.
- Do not grasp the forearm, which may pull the skin.

温石按摩

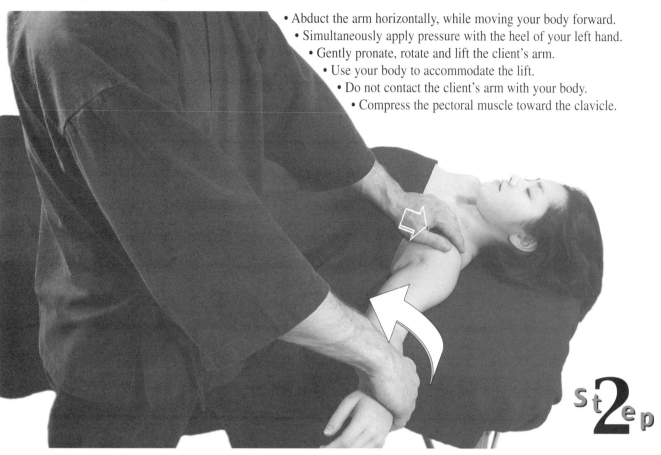

- Abduct the arm horizontally, while moving your body forward.
- Simultaneously apply pressure with the heel of your left hand.
- Gently pronate, rotate and lift the client's arm.
- Use your body to accommodate the lift.
- Do not contact the client's arm with your body.
- Compress the pectoral muscle toward the clavicle.

Step 2

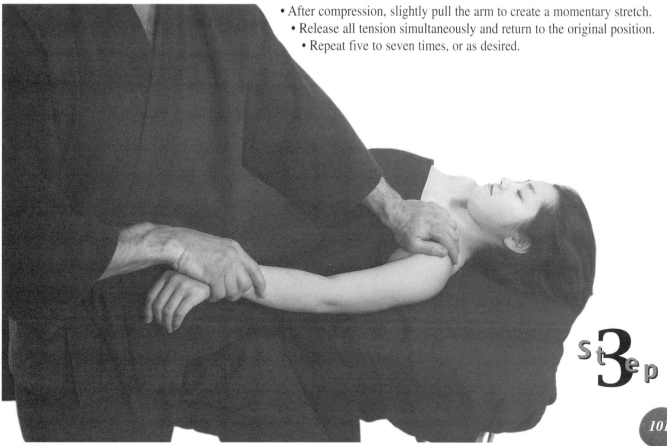

- After compression, slightly pull the arm to create a momentary stretch.
- Release all tension simultaneously and return to the original position.
- Repeat five to seven times, or as desired.

Step 3

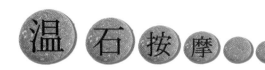

Lesson Thirty-Three

温石揉揑法
Kenbiki Technique on the Biceps

This *kenbiki* technique shares concepts with the previous technique, except the focuse is on the biceps. This technique uses light compression and small movements to accommodate the size of the muscle. In the absence of muscle tone, avoid compressing the bone and brachial artery, or omit this technique altogether. Due to the sensitivity of this area and the weight and the heat of the stone, you should apply pressure carefully. Synchronize the pressure and traction to refrain from pulling the client's skin. Use gentle movements, and if your client resists, gently shake the entire arm and repeat the movement with a smaller, more gentle range of motion.

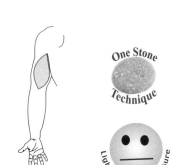

Area of Application

One Stone Technique

Light to Medium Pressure

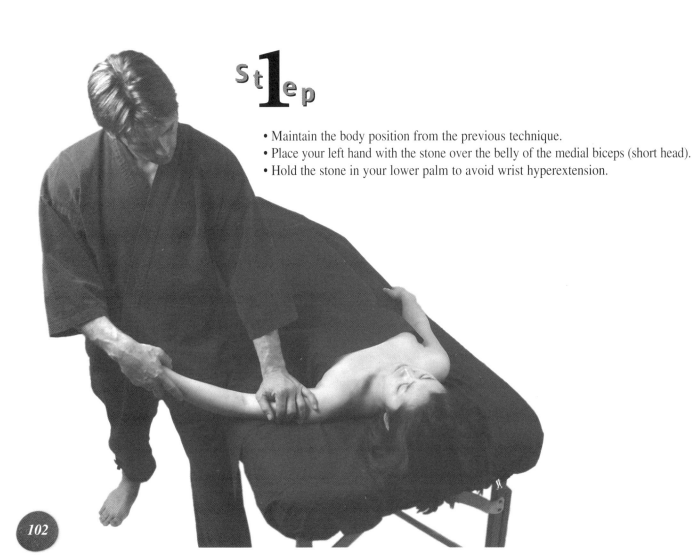

Step 1

- Maintain the body position from the previous technique.
- Place your left hand with the stone over the belly of the medial biceps (short head).
- Hold the stone in your lower palm to avoid wrist hyperextension.

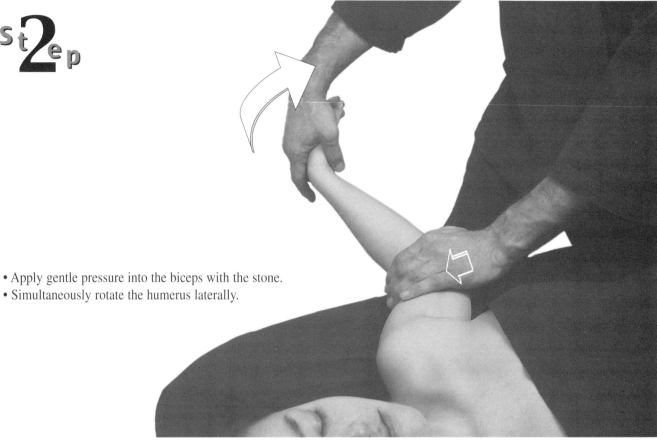

- Apply gentle pressure into the biceps with the stone.
- Simultaneously rotate the humerus laterally.

- Sustain compression with your left hand.
- Rotate the humerus medially by bringing the arm back toward your hip.
- Release all tension simultaneously and return to the original position.
- Repeat five to seven times, or as desired.

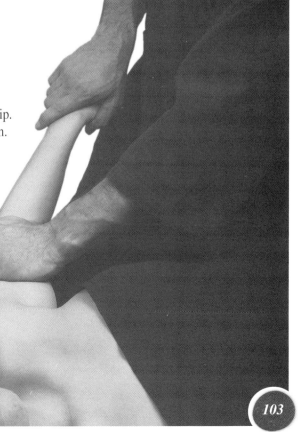

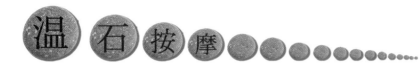

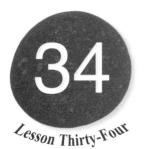

34

Lesson Thirty-Four

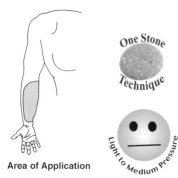

Area of Application

One Stone Technique

Light to Medium Pressure

温石揉捏法
Kneading the Flexors with Supination

This technique is very similar to the two previous techniques, and is used to reduce tension in the flexor muscles. Modern occupations require the use of computers and keyboards, which create problems, such as carpal tunnel syndrome and repetitive stress injuries. Relieving tension and reducing inflammation from the flexor muscles will significantly improve these problems. You may find that people with these occupations have extremely tight forearms, due to a lack of circulation or tense muscles and tendons. If your client is comfortable enough, you may extend their arm as in the previous technique, and lean your body weight into the table. Be careful when using your body strength, because you can easily apply significant pressure. Always apply pressure in a medial to lateral direction, because the opposite direction will not engage the muscle attachment. As with the previous lesson, this technique requires only one stone. Rotation should slow down in proportion to the depth of pressure. Do not apply pressure to the inside elbow, anterior carpal region or bony areas of the wrist.

Step 1

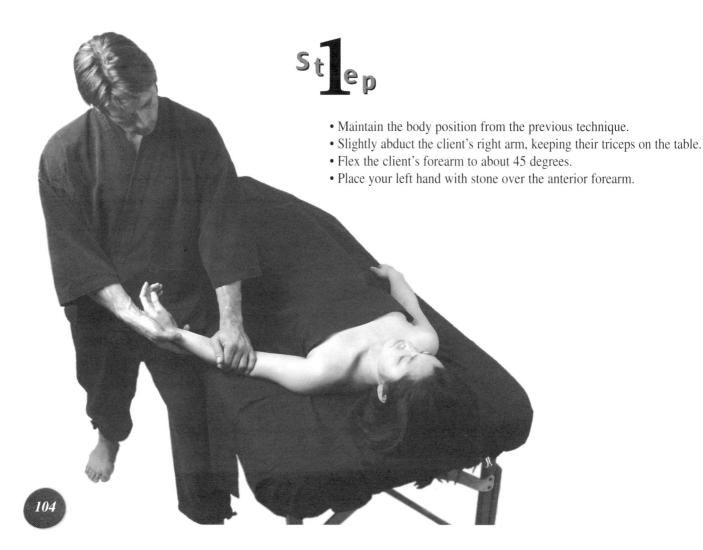

- Maintain the body position from the previous technique.
- Slightly abduct the client's right arm, keeping their triceps on the table.
- Flex the client's forearm to about 45 degrees.
- Place your left hand with stone over the anterior forearm.

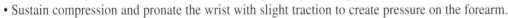

溫石按摩

Step 2

• Squeeze your fingers and stone into the forearm with gentle, even pressure.
• Simultaneously rotate the forearm laterally (away from your body).
• Sustain compression and pronate the wrist with slight traction to create pressure on the forearm.

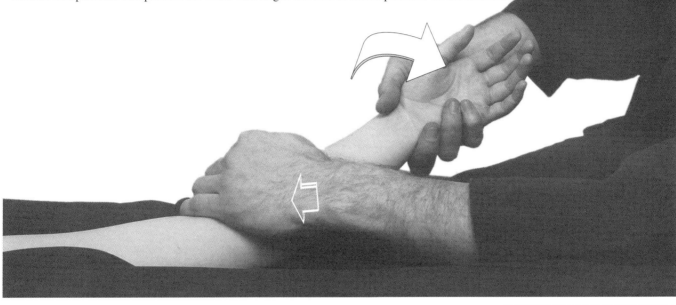

Step 3

• Release the compression and pronation.
• Repeat several times.
• Reposition distally and continue over the anterior forearm.

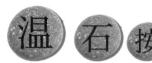 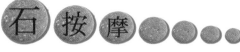

35
Lesson Thirty-Five

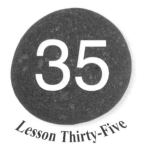

One Stone Technique

Very Light Pressure

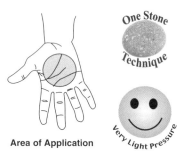

Area of Application

Gentle Compression on the Palm

Ki transfers from one meridian to another at points on the chest, hands, face and feet, so these areas are crucial for proper balance and flow of human *ki* energy. Because the hands receive more stimulation than any other region, *ki* stagnation is very rare. You may perform hot stone massage on the hands, but detailed techniques require smaller stones. The tsubo in the center of the palm is one of the gates through which energy passes in and out of the body. This tsubo point is often used in martial arts and various ancient healing arts, such as *qi gong*, to move *ki* energy and treat various conditions. The center of the palm opens energy channels that flow to all six arm meridians and central *ki* flow vessels from the internal body. Applying hot stones at the center of the palm helps open and restore the center channels. If you are interested in learning more techniques for stimulating tsubo points and meridians in the hands, please refer to *Shiatsu for the Hand*, a manual by Shogo Mochizuki.

Step 1

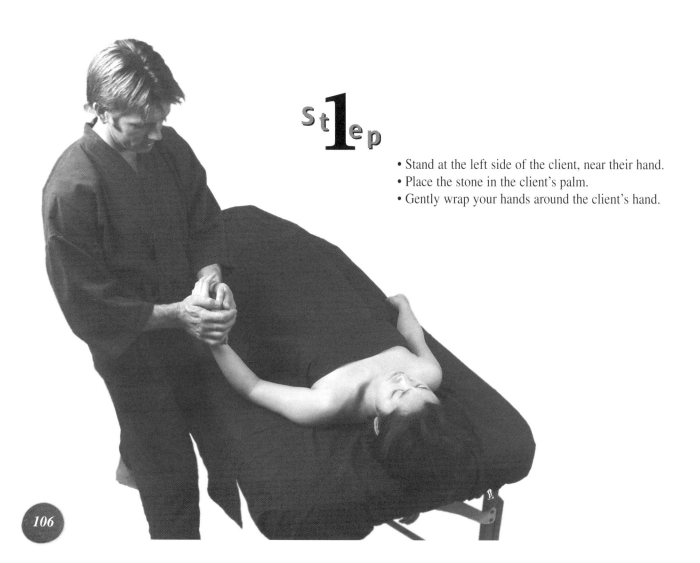

- Stand at the left side of the client, near their hand.
- Place the stone in the client's palm.
- Gently wrap your hands around the client's hand.

• Squeeze your hands together to compress the stone in the client's hand.
• As their wrist relaxes, you may add gentle rotation.
• Apply for ten to fifteen seconds.

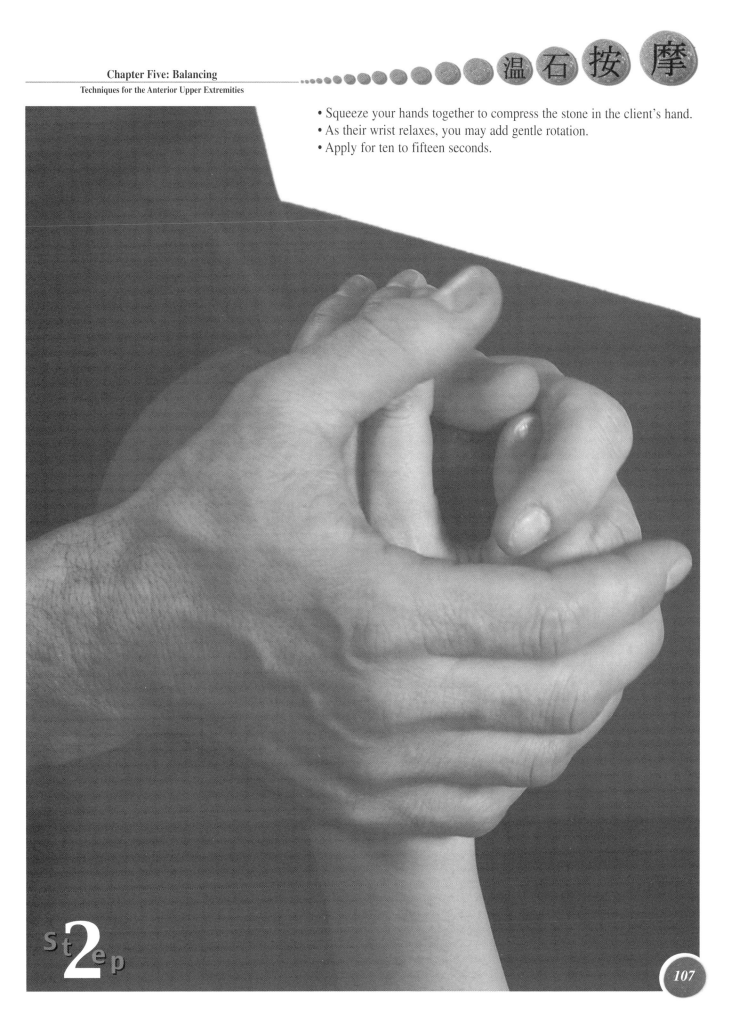

st2ep

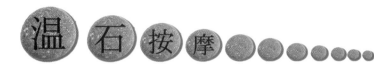

温石揉提法
Kneading the Extensors with Supination

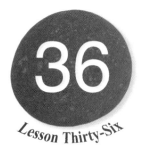

Lesson Thirty-Six

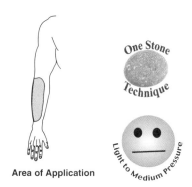

Area of Application

One Stone Technique

Light to Medium Pressure

This technique follows *ki* flow from the hand, through the posterior side of the arm, to the shoulder. If the flexors are tight while applying Lesson #34, the extensors may also be tense and will need specific attention. Due to the superficial exposure of meridians on the extensors, excessive pressure may cause latent discomfort. This technique is very similar to the *kenbiki* technique; however, you may perform small rotations if you find it difficult to apply. Adjust the diameter and pressure of your rotations to accommodate the tone of the client's extensors. If the extensors are underdeveloped, apply this technique with less pressure or very small, gentle rotations. If you are unable to avoid contacting the bones, omit rotations and only apply gentle pressure. You may continue this rotation and pressure technique over the brachioradialis and upper arm.

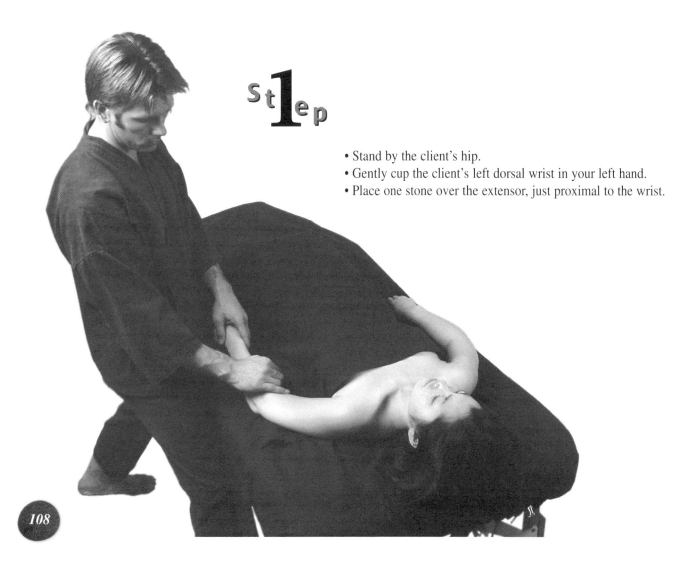

Step 1

- Stand by the client's hip.
- Gently cup the client's left dorsal wrist in your left hand.
- Place one stone over the extensor, just proximal to the wrist.

温石按摩

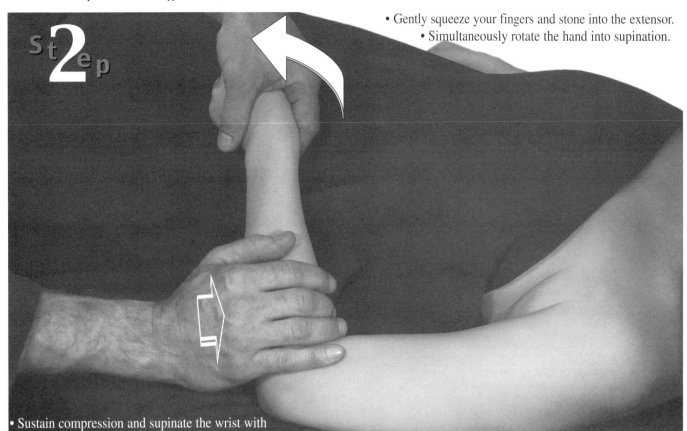

- Gently squeeze your fingers and stone into the extensor.
- Simultaneously rotate the hand into supination.

- Sustain compression and supinate the wrist with slight traction to create pressure on the forearm.

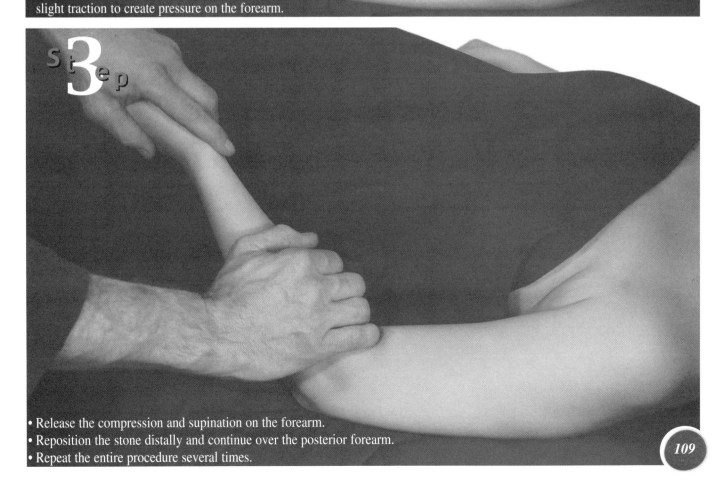

- Release the compression and supination on the forearm.
- Reposition the stone distally and continue over the posterior forearm.
- Repeat the entire procedure several times.

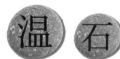
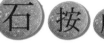
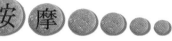

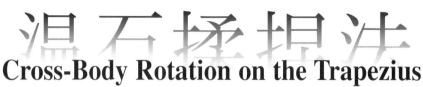

Cross-Body Rotation on the Trapezius

③⑦

Lesson Thirty-Seven

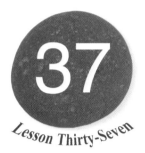

Area of Application

One Stone Technique

Medium to Heavy Pressure

The base of the neck, between the upper rhomboids, is one of the most tension-filled areas in the modern body. This technique effectively releases tension from the base of the neck, but because this technique can be stressful for the therapist, you must avoid potential low back stress. Those with existing back conditions must use extreme caution when performing this technique or omit it completely. Working on heavy-set clients may also be stressful for your body. Widen your stance to lower your body position and hook your knee under the table for stability. If your body feels extreme stress, however, you must omit this technique. For women with larger breasts, perform this technique with only one stone and one hand. Bring your elbow as close to the client's body as possible without making contact, to increase the effectiveness of this technique. Rotation comes from entire body movement, not from your hands and wrists alone.

Step 1

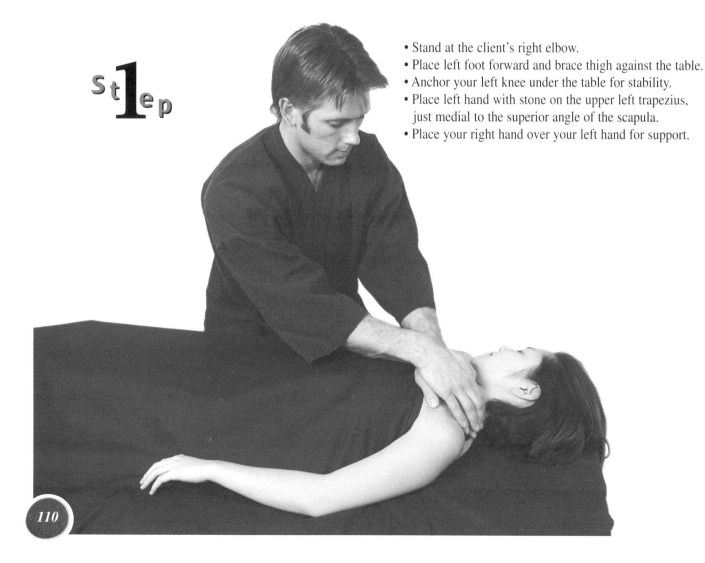

- Stand at the client's right elbow.
- Place left foot forward and brace thigh against the table.
- Anchor your left knee under the table for stability.
- Place left hand with stone on the upper left trapezius, just medial to the superior angle of the scapula.
- Place your right hand over your left hand for support.

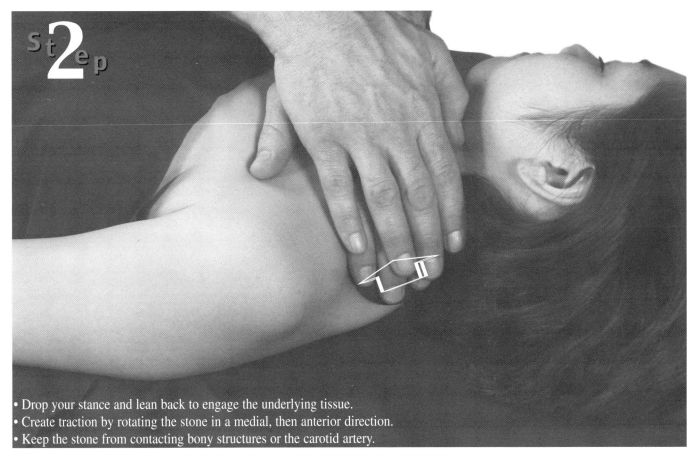

St**2**ep

- Drop your stance and lean back to engage the underlying tissue.
- Create traction by rotating the stone in a medial, then anterior direction.
- Keep the stone from contacting bony structures or the carotid artery.

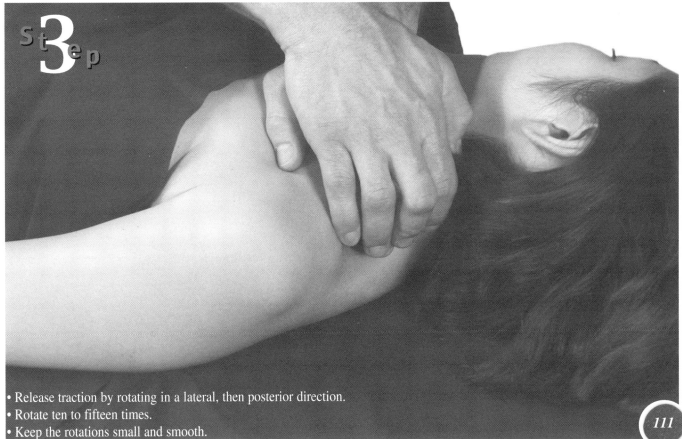

St**3**ep

- Release traction by rotating in a lateral, then posterior direction.
- Rotate ten to fifteen times.
- Keep the rotations small and smooth.

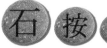 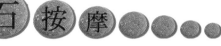

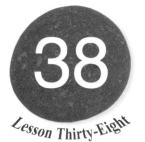

38

Lesson Thirty-Eight

Two Stone
Technique

Very Light Pressure

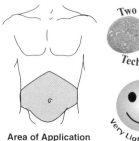
Area of Application

温石軽擦法
Light Stroking Over the Abdomen

When you finish massaging the arms and shoulders, begin *anpuku* therapy by applying gentle strokes over the abdomen. This two-stone technique calms the internal organs to restore balance to the *hara*. *Anpuku* is traditionally applied from the right side of the table, and therapists do not switch sides during treatment. *Hara* is the Japanese word for "abdomen," and in traditional Japanese medicine, the *hara* is the most important part of the human body. All illnesses are believed to originate from a *hara* imbalance. *Anpuku* therapy has been traced back to the fifth century in Japan, when many surgical procedures were not available. *Anpuku* therapists were called *hara tori*, and were considered the highest ranking medical professionals for many centuries. *Anpuku* therapy is difficult to master; therefore, limited treatment was only available to imperial families and the warrior class. This is a good time to use a fresh set of stones, but be sure the temperature of the stones is suitable for your client. We recommend that you always apply *anpuku* therapy techniques over sheets, because this area can be very sensitive to heat. Remove bolsters from beneath the legs during all *anpuku* treatments.

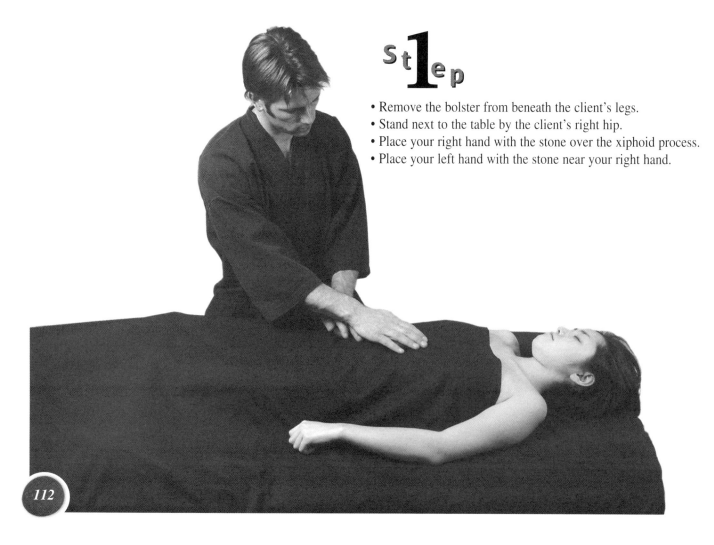

Step 1

- Remove the bolster from beneath the client's legs.
- Stand next to the table by the client's right hip.
- Place your right hand with the stone over the xiphoid process.
- Place your left hand with the stone near your right hand.

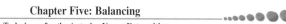

温石按摩

step 2

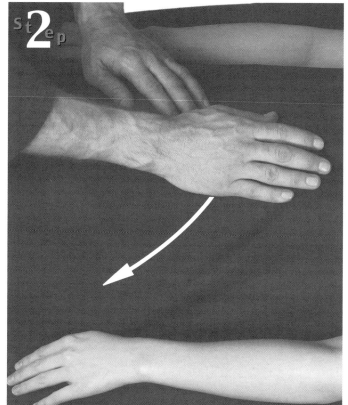

- Stroke your left hand laterally along the edge of the rib cage.
- As left hand finishes, place right hand below the xiphoid process.

step 3

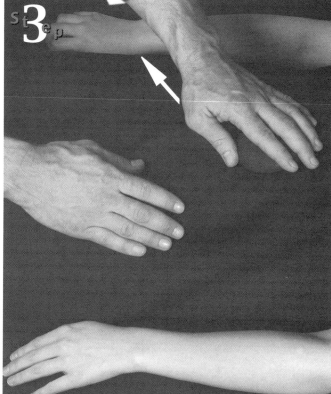

- Stroke your right hand laterally along the edge of the rib cage.
- Continue smooth, slow strokes.

step 4

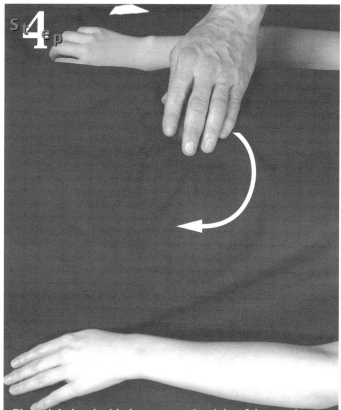

- Place right hand with the stone to the right of the navel.
- Begin clockwise, circular strokes around the navel.

step 5

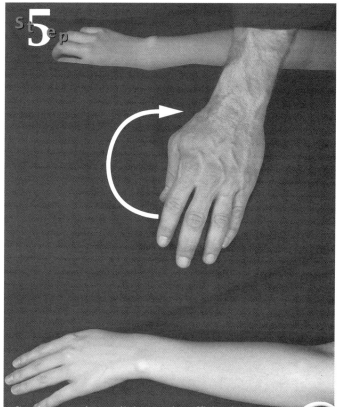

- Continue rotating until the area is sufficiently warmed.
- Apply ten to twenty rotations.

113

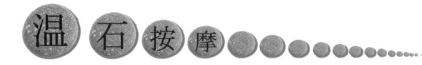

温石揉捏法
Anpuku Kneading with Four Stones

39

Lesson Thirty-Nine

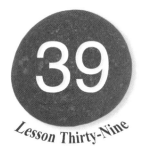

Four Stone

Technique

Medium to Heavy Pressure

Area of Application

Continue applying *anpuku* therapy to the *hara* by kneading around the navel. Use circular kneading to distribute pressure throughout the four stones and to gently massage the Small Intestine. In traditional Asian medicine, the Small Intestine is very important, because it absorbs energy from food, which is considered to be earth essence. Efficient food energy absorption is essential for human function. Improper small intestine function can result in low energy, chronic fatigue and other energy imbalances, which create problems with human function. You should only apply this circular movement during exhalation; however, as your client becomes more comfortable, you may apply two rotations per exhalation. Do not let the stones contact each other during this treatment, because the striking noise can be distracting for you and your client.

Step 1

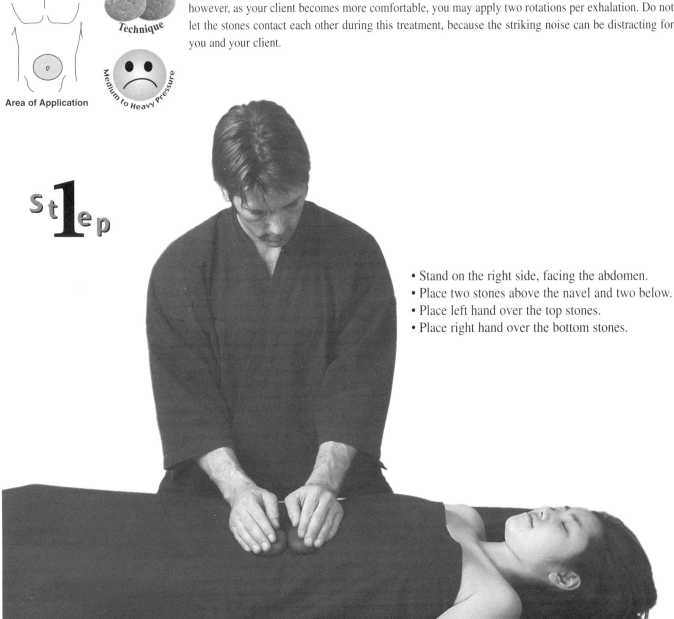

• Stand on the right side, facing the abdomen.
• Place two stones above the navel and two below.
• Place left hand over the top stones.
• Place right hand over the bottom stones.

温 石 按 摩

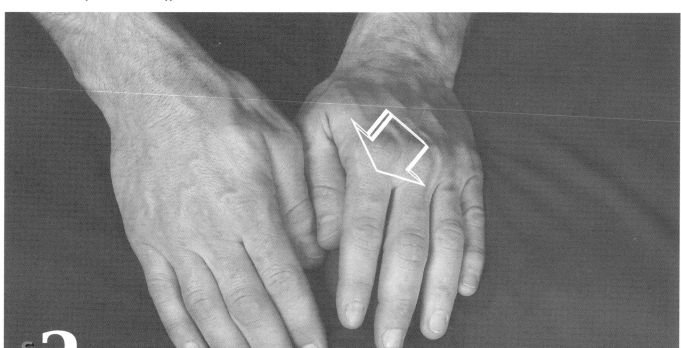

St2ep

• Apply gentle pressure toward the navel with the heel of your left hand.
• Apply gentle pressure toward the navel with your left fingertips.

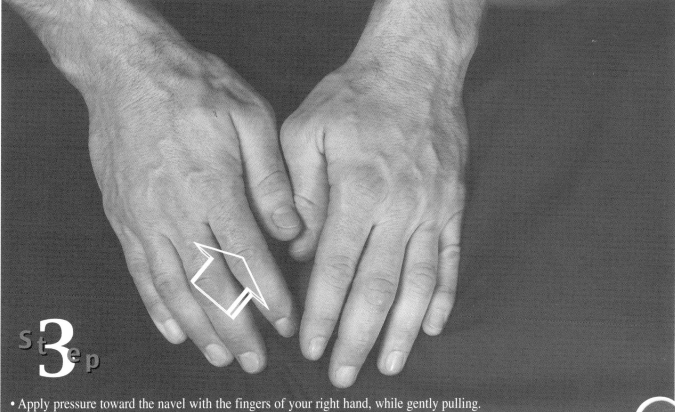

St3ep

• Apply pressure toward the navel with the fingers of your right hand, while gently pulling.
• Apply pressure toward the navel with the heel of your right hand, while gently pushing; repeat 10-15 times.

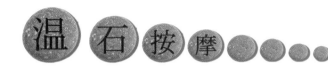

温石圧迫法
Activating Tsubo on the Conception Vessel

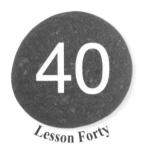

Lesson Forty

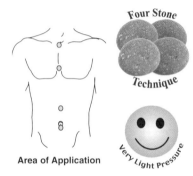

Area of Application

Four Stone Technique

Very Light Pressure

Anpuku therapy is an independent therapy and is one of the most difficult to master. There are hundreds of *anpuku* techniques, but the three we cover will be most beneficial to your clients. This is a continuation of the previous technique, so place the four stones that were once over the abdomen over the Conception Vessel tsubo. The lower tsubo, *chu kan* and *ki kai*, are two of the ten most important tsubo on the human body for maintaining health and longevity. Moxabustion, which is heat therapy, is the most effective way to treat these tsubo points, so hot stones are also very therapeutic. Stimulating these two tsubo points with hot stones will create a moxabustion effect and will restore balance to the human body. The bottom stones balance the entire digestive system, while the top stones balance heart and respiratory conditions. If the stones don't naturally stay on the tsubo points, you may need to manually secure their position. This is one of the most calming and balancing stages of the entire massage, so remain calm and centered to facilitate your client's relaxation.

Step 1

• Maintain the body position from the previous technique.
• Place one stone over *dan chu* (Conception Vessel-17).

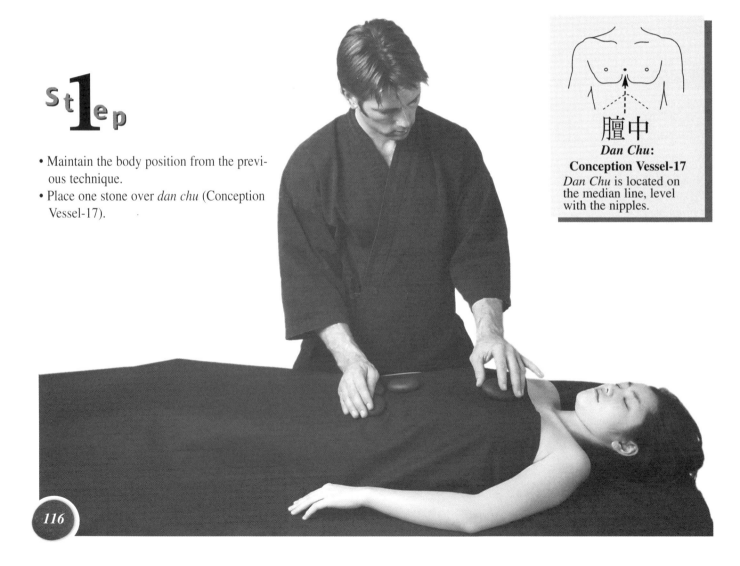

膻中
***Dan Chu*:**
Conception Vessel-17
Dan Chu is located on the median line, level with the nipples.

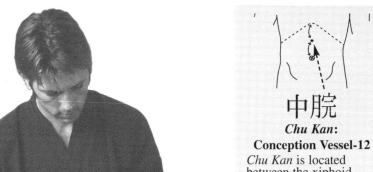

St2ep

- Place another stone over *chu kan* (Conception Vessel-12).

中脘
Chu Kan:
Conception Vessel-12
Chu Kan is located between the xiphoid process and the navel on the median line.

St3ep

- Place another stone over *sen ki* (Conception Vessel-21) with your left hand.
- Simultanously move a stone to *ki kai* (Conception Vessel-6) with your right hand and hold for 20-30 seconds.
- Gently and quietly remove all stones.

璇璣
Sen Ki:
Conception Vessel-21
Sen Ki is located on the median line, level with the first rib.

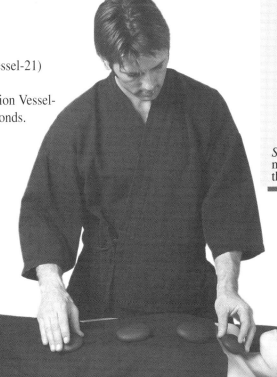

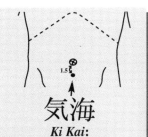

気海
Ki Kai:
Conception Vessel-6
Ki Kai is located one and a half thumb-widths inferior to the navel on the median line.

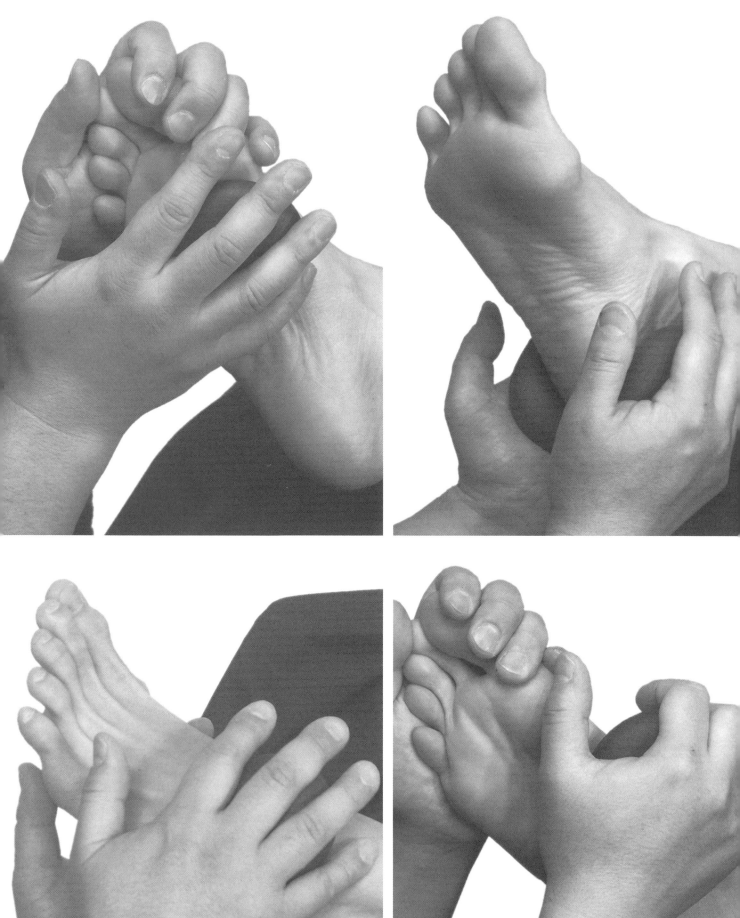

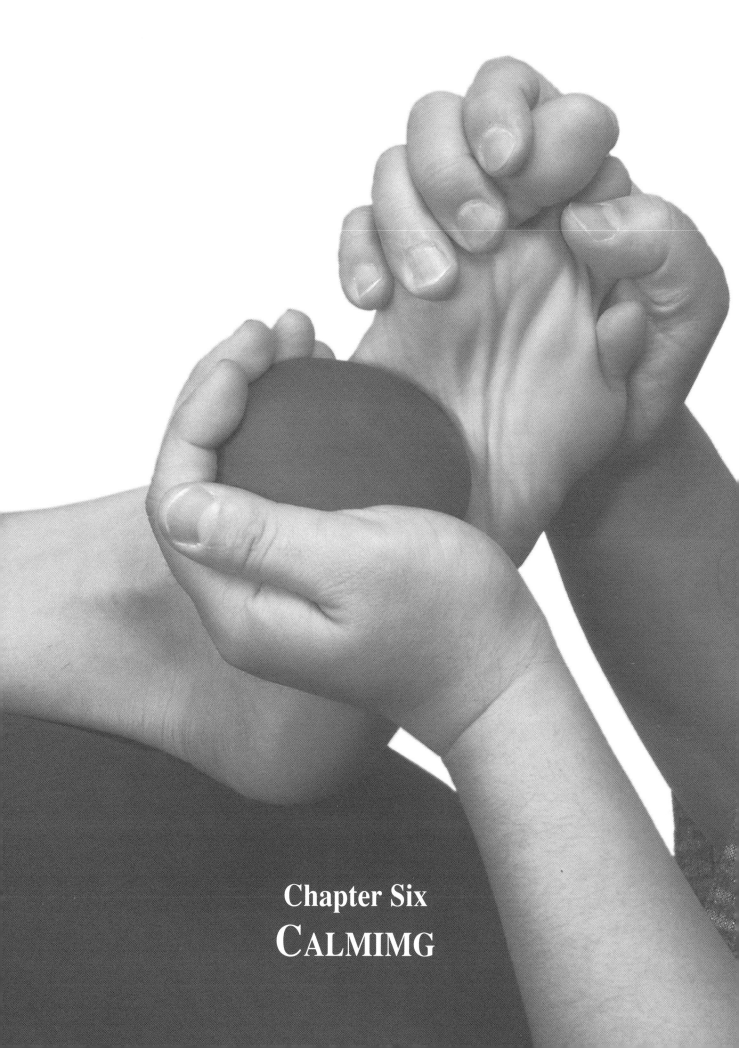

Chapter Six
CALMIMG

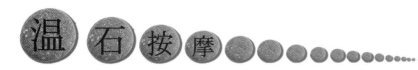
Chapter Six
CALMING
Techniques for the Anterior Lower Extremities

In this chapter, we present ten techniques for the anterior lower extremities. The techniques in this chapter represent water, the element that signifies calming. After *yin* and calming *anpuku* therapy, slowly integrate more active *yang* techniques, while keeping the treatment calm and harmonious. Ease into anterior leg and foot treatment without being too aggressive.

We demonstrate all of the techniques in this chapter on the left side of the body. After you have treated the entire left side, reverse your hand and body position to massage the right side. Practice these techniques on both sides of the body, but apply them all to one side before the other. Western massage therapists are often taught to work from the tip of the extremities in toward the heart. Asian bodywork, however, works from the center of the body out toward the extremities.

The anterior thigh can often be very invasive for clients, and if the draping becomes a problem, you should apply these techniques over the sheets. Otherwise, your client should be properly draped in all areas, except the one on which you are working. If necessary, use a blanket to ensure that your client is warm and comfortable.

When applying foot massage in the supine position, place additional bolsters beneath the calves to raise the client's foot to your seated chest level and reduce the angle of your wrist.

The first techniques work on the anterior and lateral legs, where the Stomach and Gall Bladder meridians are located. These two meridians assist the Spleen and Bladder meridians in purifying the blood and lymphatic system. With the client in the supine position, you can also address the Kidney and Bladder meridians, which requires more extensive knowledge of Asian bodywork and will be covered in *Shiatsu with Hot Stones*.

温石按摩

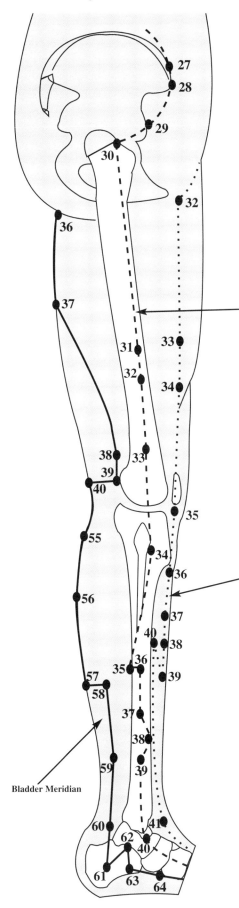

Bladder Meridian

Meridians in the Legs

Of the six meridians that run through the legs, the three *yin* meridians run through the medial portion of the legs, were explained in Chapter Four. The three *yang* meridians in the lateral legs actually begin around the eyes. The Bladder meridian, which was explained in Chapter Three, goes over the back of the head, along the spine, through the center of the posterior legs and ends in the fourth toe. The Gall Bladder meridian runs through the side of the head, through the side of the torso, down the lateral side of the legs, over the iliotibial tract and through the lateral portion of the legs to the fifth toe. The Stomach meridian runs down the front of the face and throat, over the breasts, down the anterior center of the legs, over the tibialis anterior and ends at the second toe.

Please note that when an internal organ is capitalized, it refers to the Asian form of the organ. Asian and Western ideas of internal organ function are often quite different. This book briefly introduces meridians, but for further information about meridians, tsubo and their functions, please refer to *Shiatsu for the Hand* and *Shiatsu for the Foot*.

Gall Bladder Meridian

The Gall Bladder meridian is known as the "Palace of the Central and Upright," because it makes both physical and psychological decisions for human function. The Gall Bladder also stores *Tan Ju*, the most pure liquid in the human body, which is similar to the Western understanding of bile. The Gall Bladder is closely related to the Liver, which assists in deep thinking and planning. Together, the Gall Bladder and Liver become the foundation of our psychological activity. If the Liver and Gall Bladder both become irregular or an imbalance develops between the two, one of the two will be unable to make decisions and will cease productivity. The Gall Bladder has a close connection to the shoulder, the side of the head and the side of the body. It is also closely connected to diseases in the feet, and a loss of mobility in the legs or lower limbs. Headache, tinnitus, dizziness, neurological pain, excessive sweating and pain in the ovaries are all often related to a Gall Bladder imbalance. A bitter taste in the mouth is another indication that the Gall Bladder is compromised in some manner.

Stomach Meridian

The Stomach incorporates several parts of the digestive system, including the mouth, tongue, esophagus and the stomach itself. The main function of the stomach is somewhat close to Western physiology; however, Asian medicine believes that the stomach has its own intelligence. The stomach first examines food and rejects food that is of poor quality. It then begins the digestion process by breaking down food and bringing it to the correct temperature for digestion. These functions have lead the Stomach to be known as the "Palace of Food Essence" and "Sea of Nutrients."

The Stomach and Spleen work closely together within the Earth element. The Stomach prepares food for digestion and the Spleen transforms it into usable nutrients, before transporting them to the internal organs. Spleen dysfunction affects the Stomach in various ways. For example, during menstruation, some women lose their appetites and have poor digestion. People who are under heavy stress also develop poor digestion. Conversely, conditions in the Stomach also affect the Spleen. If the stomach is unable to digest food, the Spleen will be unable to transform and distribute nutrients.

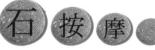
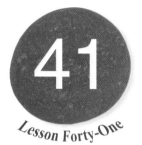

41

Lesson Forty-One

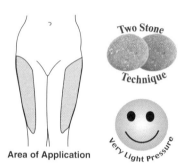

Area of Application

Two Stone Technique

Very Light Pressure

Light Stroking Over the Anterior Thigh

Begin working on the lower extremities by applying smooth, light strokes with a fresh set of warm stones. To make this stroke as smooth and comfortable as possible, place a bolster behind your client's knees and only stroke their upper thigh. The bolster and the bony surface of the lower leg make it extremely difficult to apply a continuous and comfortable stroke along the entire leg. Therefore, it is best to work only the upper thigh during this application. The upper thigh, especially the medial portion, is extremely sensitive to temperature. To accommodate this sensitivity, stroke quickly and continuously until the stones have cooled or work through a sheet. Allow the stones to cool to an appropriate temperature before proceeding to the following techniques. Never apply deep, slow, localized techniques with stones that are too hot for your client.

Step 1

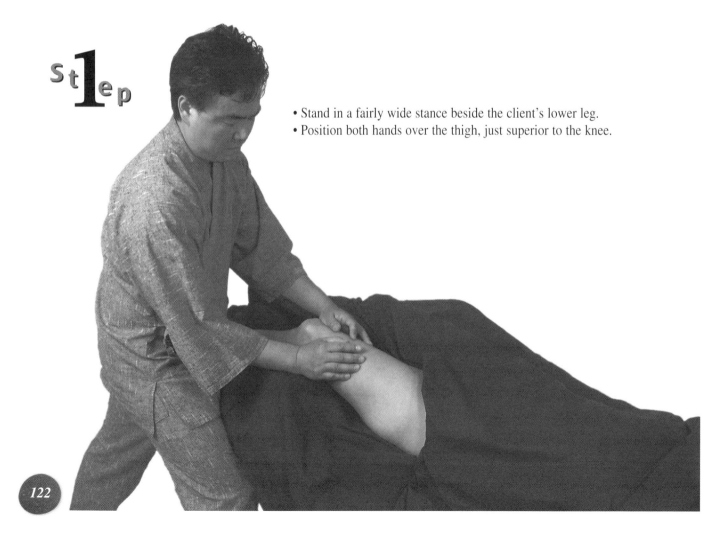

- Stand in a fairly wide stance beside the client's lower leg.
- Position both hands over the thigh, just superior to the knee.

温 石 按

• Simultaneously stroke both hands inferiorly.
• As you approach the hips, reposition laterally, as to not infringe upon the groin region.

ˢᵗ**2**ₑₚ

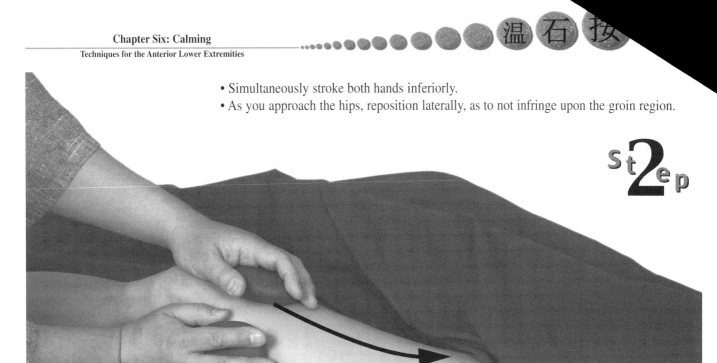

• Once you reach the lateral hip, return along the same path to complete the stroke.
• Stroke ten to fifteen times, or as desired.
• Keep your elbows in and your shoulders dropped and relaxed.

ˢᵗ**3**ₑₚ

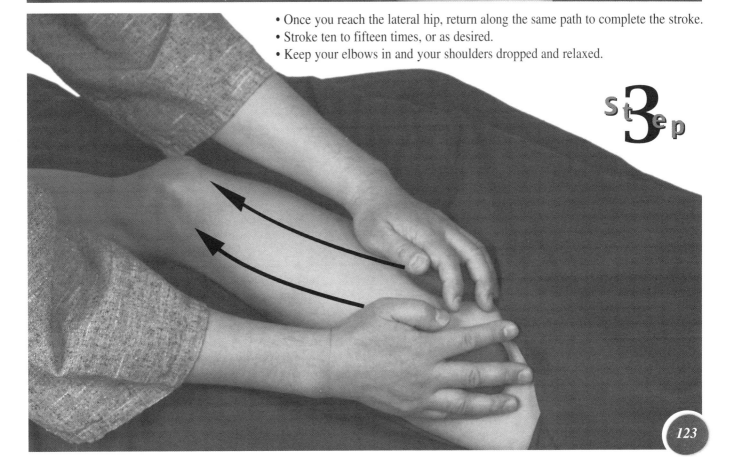

123

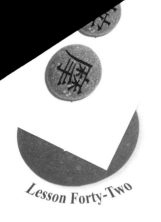

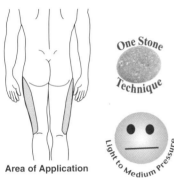

Lesson Forty-Two

Area of Application

One Stone Technique

Light to Medium Pressure

温石揉提法
Rotation Along the Gall Bladder Meridian

Many people accumulate significant tension in their hips and greater trochanter. This technique is excellent for reducing tension around the greater trochanter, hips, low back and lateral legs. This technique is best applied with the client lying in the side position; however, it will also work in the supine position. When applying this technique in the supine position, gently rotate the client's torso by adducting their femur across their body as far as comfortably possible. This position allows you to easily access the Gall Bladder meridian without stressing your wrists. Lower your stance to facilitate a safe and effective wrist angle. When adjusting your body position, focus primarily on your wrist angle, as well as proper elbow and shoulder alignment. Applying this technique without wrist stress may be slightly awkward and uncomfortable. In this case, an uncomfortable body position does not necessarily mean that it's incorrect. Continue and apply rotation, but do not maintain an uncomfortable position for extended periods of time. Apply this rotation along the posterior edge of the IT band, from the greater trochanter to the patella.

Step 1

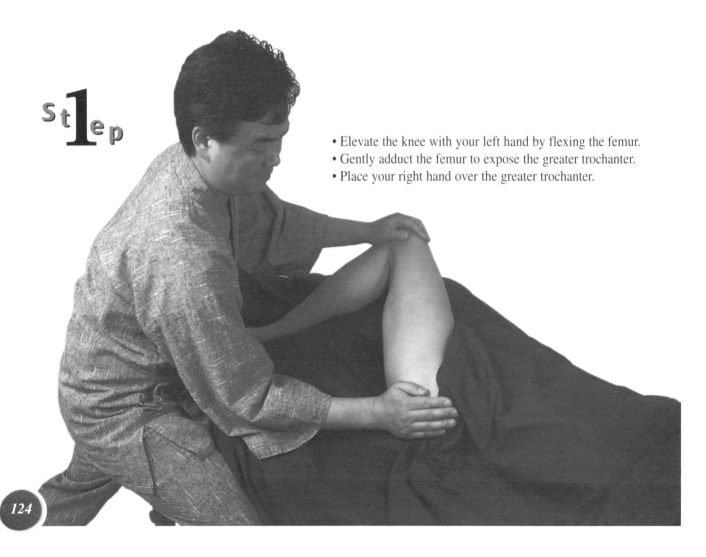

• Elevate the knee with your left hand by flexing the femur.
• Gently adduct the femur to expose the greater trochanter.
• Place your right hand over the greater trochanter.

• Apply pressure with your right hand to engage the underlying tissue.
• Rotate in a superior, anterior, inferior and posterior direction.
• Repeat five to ten rotations.

Step 2

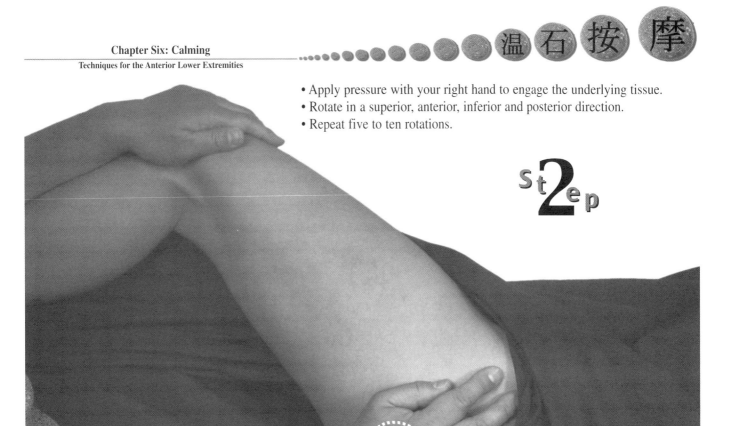

• Continue rotating as you gradually reposition about a palm-width inferior.
• Repeat five to ten more rotations.
• Work your way along the IT band until you reach the superior patella.

Step 3

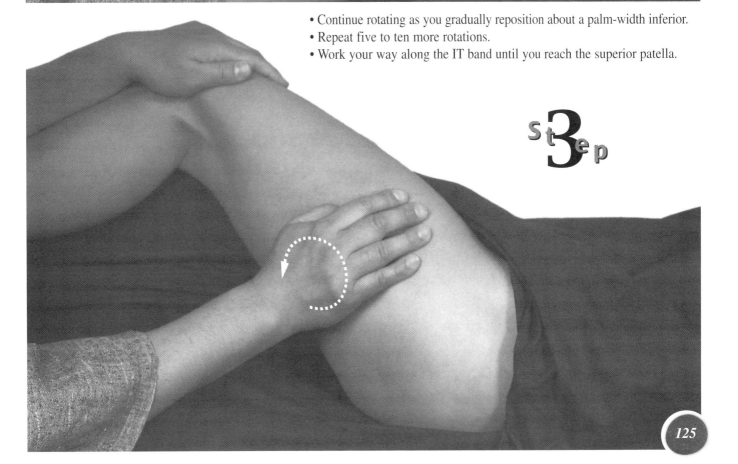

125

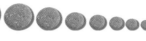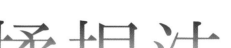

温石揉提法
Rotation Over the Lateral Thigh

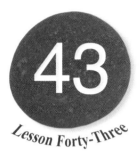
Area of Application

One Stone Technique

Light to Medium Pressure

Continue using the rotation technique from Lesson # 42 to reduce lateral thigh tension. If you are familiar with sports massage, you know that this technique can effectively tune weak muscles and reduce tension. Due to the volume of the thigh muscle, this technique can stimulate tired muscles or relax over-stimulated muscles. Despite the significant size of the thigh muscle, you should use only minimal pressure for this technique. Applying this type of rotation to such a large muscle group can increase blood flow, which removes metabolites stored in the tissue from overuse or poor circulation. The gentle femur movement included in this *kenbiki* technique also has a positive effect on sacroiliac dysfunction. Finger placement is inconsequential when applying this technique on the lower thigh; however, when working the upper thigh, keep your fingers parallel to the client's body and maintain a safe wrist angle. Achieve a proper wrist angle by lowering your stance and keeping your elbows close to your body.

Step 1

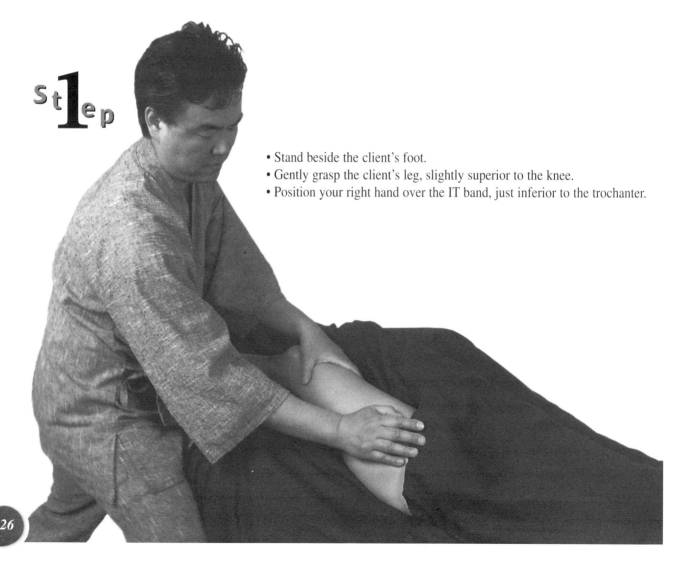

- Stand beside the client's foot.
- Gently grasp the client's leg, slightly superior to the knee.
- Position your right hand over the IT band, just inferior to the trochanter.

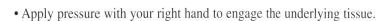 温石按摩

- Apply pressure with your right hand to engage the underlying tissue.
- Rotate in a superior, anterior, inferior and posterior direction.
- Repeat five to ten rotations.

St**2**ep

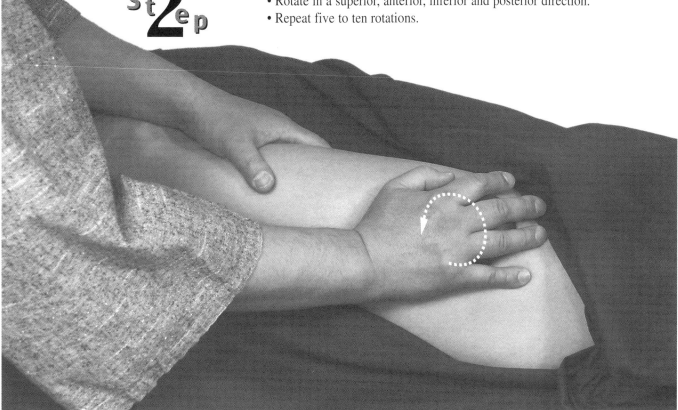

St**3**ep

- Continue rotating as you gradually reposition about one palm-width inferior.
- Repeat five to ten more rotations.
- Work your way along the IT band until you reach the superior patella.

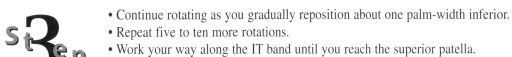

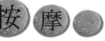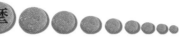

44
Lesson Forty-Four

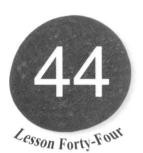
Area of Application

One Stone Technique

Light to Medium Pressure

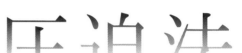
Gentle Pressure Along the Sartorius

Massage the medial thigh carefully, as it is often sensitive to aggressive applications. You may apply rotation, but slow, subtle pressure without rotation is less invasive. If your client's sensitivity permits further manipulation, apply rotation in a superior, anterior, inferior, then posterior direction. Do not depend entirely upon your rotating hand for pressure. Instead, the force behind this rotation comes from moving the client's knee into your rotating hand to compress the underlying tissues into the stone. Moving the entire leg greatly enhances the therapeutic benefits of this technique and minimizes therapist effort. To apply this technique correctly, gently rock the client's entire leg, while slightly moving your body to apply smooth, continuous pressure.

Step 1

• Stand by the client's left knee in a wide stance with right foot forward.
• Place your right hand just superior to the client's knee for stability.
• Place your left hand over the superior attachment of the sartorius, just inferior to the anterior superior iliac spine.

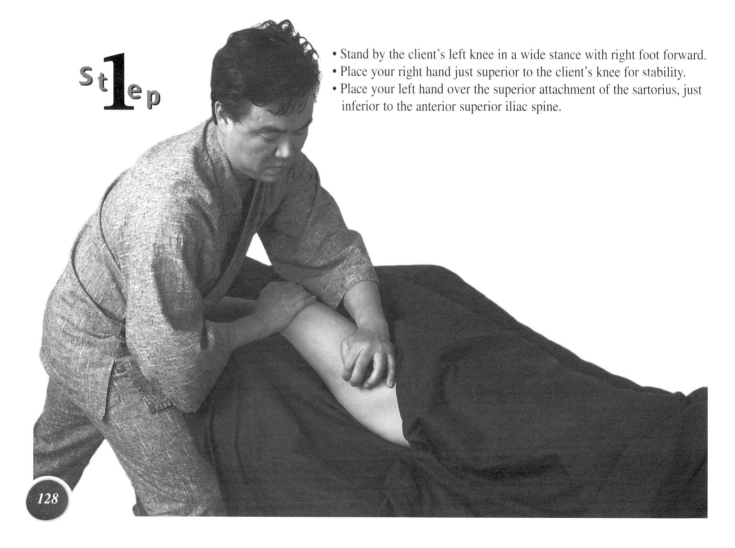

Step 2

- Apply gentle pressure with your right hand to engage the underlying tissue, and move the leg medially to facilitate the pressure.
- Repeat two to three applications.

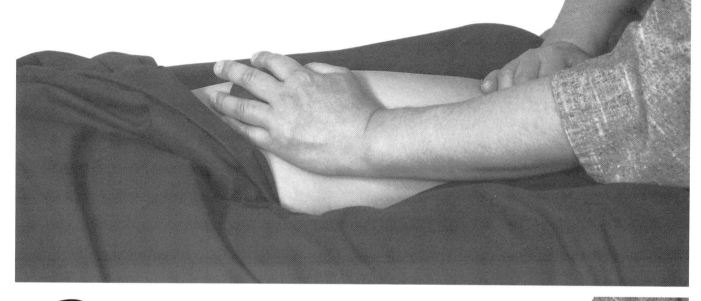

Step 3

- Reposition about one hand-width inferior.
- Repeat two to three more applications of pressure.
- Work medially along the sartorius until you reach it's inferior attachment at the knee.

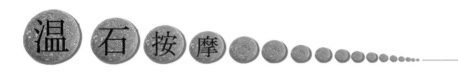

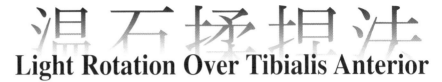

温石揉提法
Light Rotation Over Tibialis Anterior

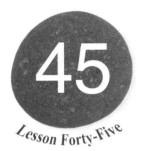
Lesson Forty-Five

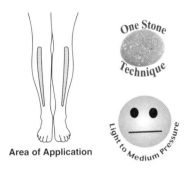
Area of Application

One Stone Technique

Light to Medium Pressure

The lower anterior leg and shin are never easy places to massage, and stones make it even more difficult. Avoiding contact with the bone can be especially challenging in this area, but clients with a well-developed tibialis anterior often have less problems. If your client's tibialis anterior is too small to avoid contact with the bone, however, you should omit this technique. This may be a good time to change to a fresh set of stones. If you do change stones, apply light strokes to acclimate the temperature before applying rotation. The tibialis anterior is often extremely tight. Digging deeply into this area may leave your client's legs extremely sore, so avoid overworking this muscle. It is important to note that this is a one-stone technique.

Step 1

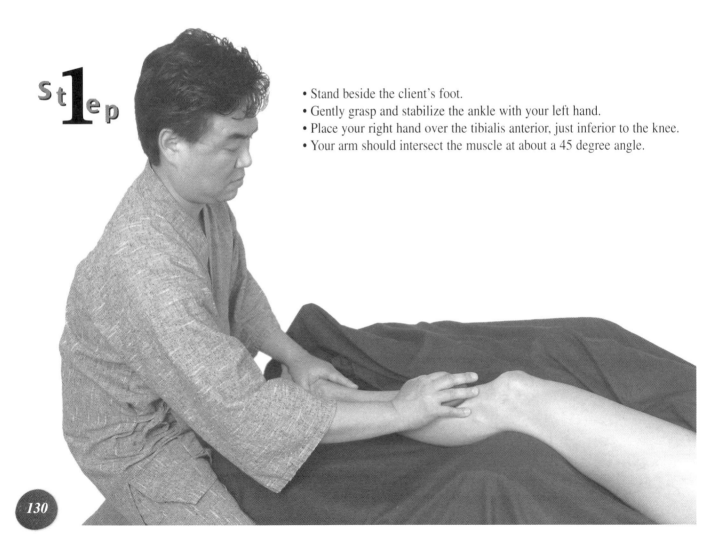

- Stand beside the client's foot.
- Gently grasp and stabilize the ankle with your left hand.
- Place your right hand over the tibialis anterior, just inferior to the knee.
- Your arm should intersect the muscle at about a 45 degree angle.

温石按摩

Step 2

- Apply pressure with your right hand to engage the underlying tissue.
- Apply small rotations in a superior, medial, inferior and lateral direction.
- Repeat five to seven rotations.

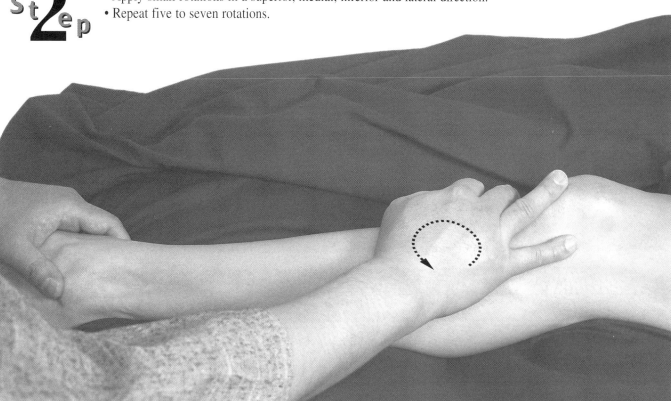

Step 3

- Continue rotating as you gradually reposition a hand-width inferior.
- Gradually work your way along the anterior tibialis until you reach the malleolus.

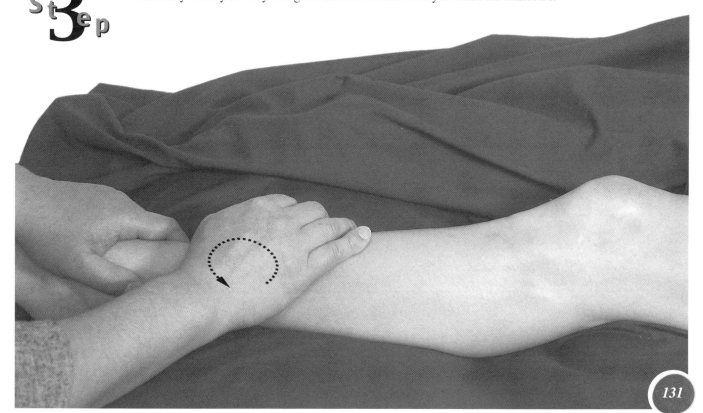

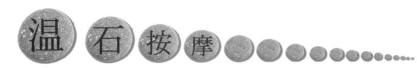

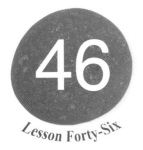

46

Lesson Forty-Six

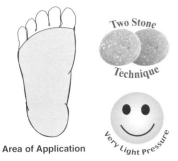

Area of Application

Two Stone

Technique

Very Light Pressure

温石軽擦法
Stroking the Foot with Two Stones

The next five lessons demonstrate Japanese Hot Stone Massage for the feet. Foot massage will add a nice, soothing touch to your treatment. Because the dorsal foot has a very dense bone structure, you should never apply heavy pressure. If this technique is too uncomfortable for your client, omit it altogether. Check the client's foot condition before beginning the massage to prevent stone contamination. If your client has athlete's foot or another condition for which massage is contraindicated, work through a sheet or other protective barrier. You can compensate for the typically moist condition of the feet by sprinkling powder on them or working through a sheet. Again, adjust your position as necessary to maintain a safe, effective wrist angle.

St1ep

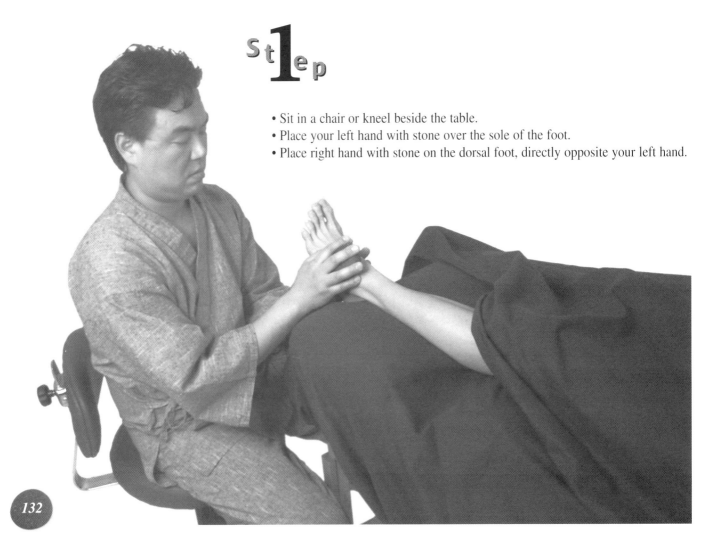

- Sit in a chair or kneel beside the table.
- Place your left hand with stone over the sole of the foot.
- Place right hand with stone on the dorsal foot, directly opposite your left hand.

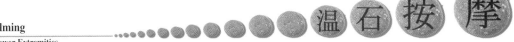

温石按摩

Step 2

• Stroke distally toward the toes with both hands simultaneously.

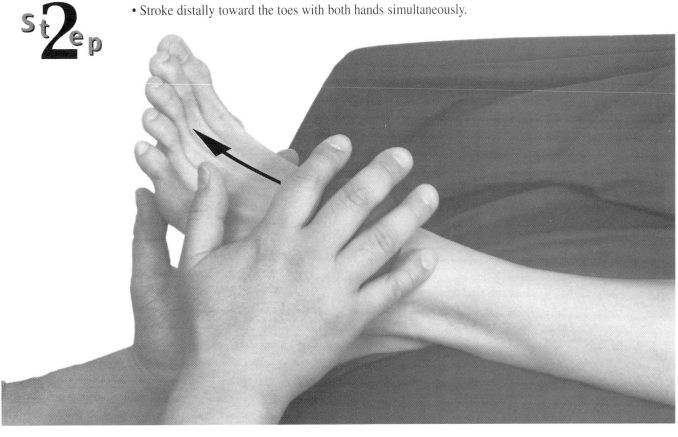

Step 3

• Upon reaching the metatarsophalangeal joints, reverse the stroke and return to the starting position.
• Repeat ten to fifteen strokes.

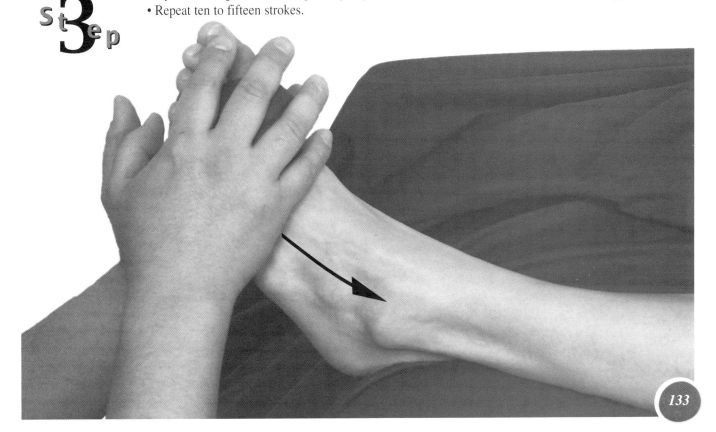

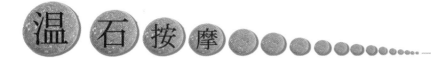

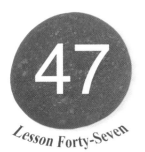

温石軽擦法
Circular Stroking on the Arch

After you warm the entire foot, stroke over the arch in a circular motion with one stone. The transition to this lesson from the previous technique is very important. While stroking with your left hand, remove your right hand and stone. Then, gently grasp the dorsal foot with your right hand for stability and stroke in a circular direction with your left hand. Cradle the stone in your fingers as you apply light strokes, but when applying deeper strokes into the arch, you must hold the stone in your palm to prevent finger hyperextension. Performing this technique at the foot of the table could lead to wrist hyperextension. To apply this technique without jeopardizing your wrist angle, sit by the corner of the massage table at a 45 degree angle. This position decreases wrist angle and creates smoother movements. Use your body position to accommodate the inversion or eversion of your client's feet and to prevent wrist hyperextension. Many foot massage techniques require you to precisely adjust your body mechanics; using a chair with wheels will allow you to make these adjustments quickly and easily.

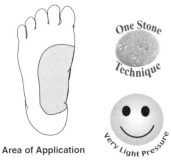

Area of Application

One Stone Technique

Very Light Pressure

St**1**ep

- Grasp the foot with your right hand.
- Position your left hand with stone on the ball of the foot.

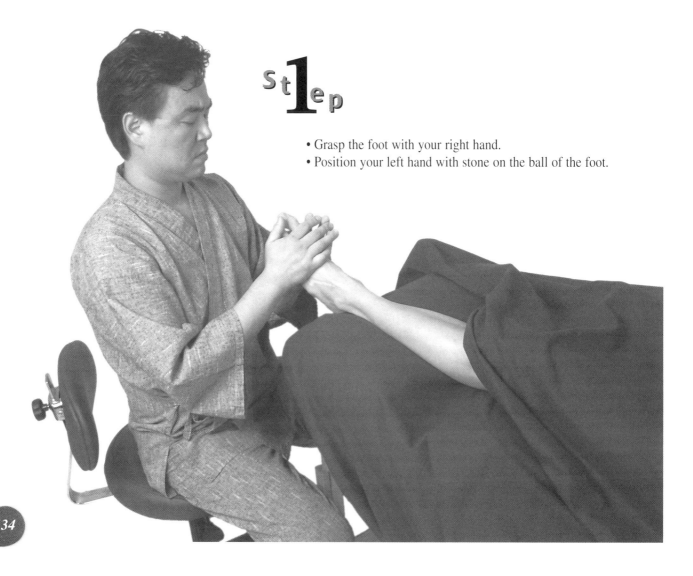

St2ep

- The diameter of this rotation spans the entire arch.
- Begin rotating in a lateral, then proximal direction.
- Avoid wrist hyperextension during this application.

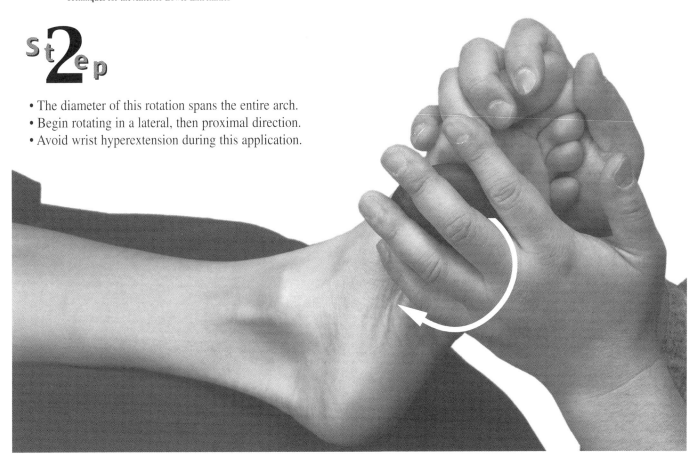

St3ep

- Continue rotating in a medial, then distal direction.
- Repeat ten to fifteen rotations.

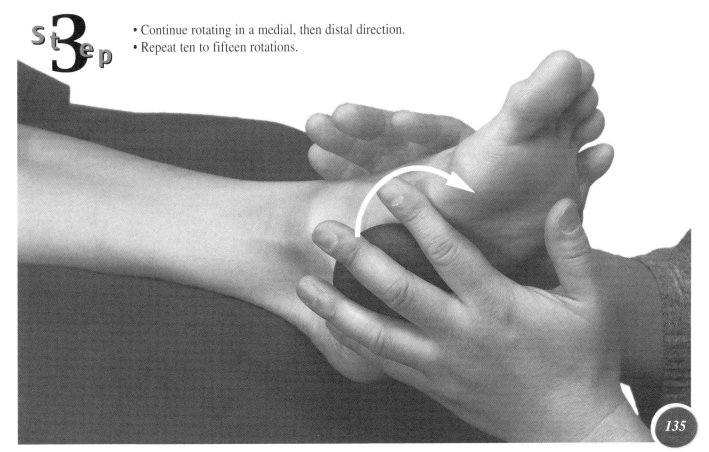

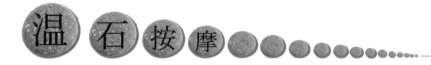

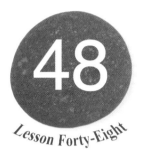

Lesson Forty-Eight

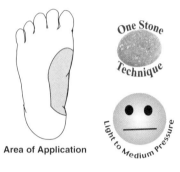

Area of Application

One Stone Technique

Light to Medium Pressure

温石揉捏法
Rotation on the Arch with One Stone

Sit at a forty-five degree angle in relation to your client's foot, with their foot raised to your approximate chest level. In *Zoku Shin Do*, traditional Japanese foot massage, the foot is compressed into the treating hand like a tool. The hand used for treatment is stabilized, and movement comes from the elbow and shoulder. The two points of movement—compressing the foot into the applying hand and simultaneously stabilizing that hand—provide adequate pressure to sustain a therapeutic level.

Do not stress your client's knee or ankle while inverting their foot for this technique. When applying this technique, you must find the safest body position for your wrist angle. Your body position should ensure that your hand and wrist are on the same parallel plane as the sole of the foot. As you knead the foot, cradle your elbow and upper arm against your body. Keep your shoulders and elbows dropped and relaxed throughout this application. As you move proximally during this technique, evert the foot, apply tension to the arch and accommodate the movement.

Step 1

• Gently grasp the foot with your right hand.
• Position your left hand with stone on the ball of the foot.

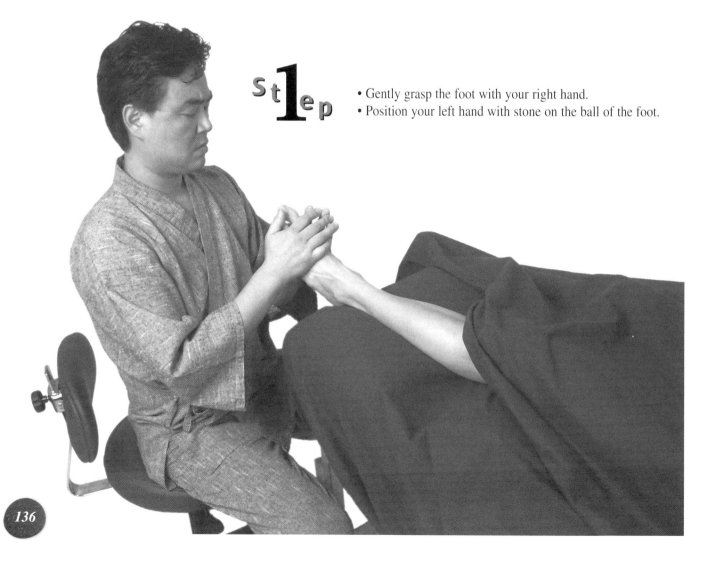

136

Step 2

- Gently compress the stone into the arch.
- Apply small rotations in a proximal, then medial direction.

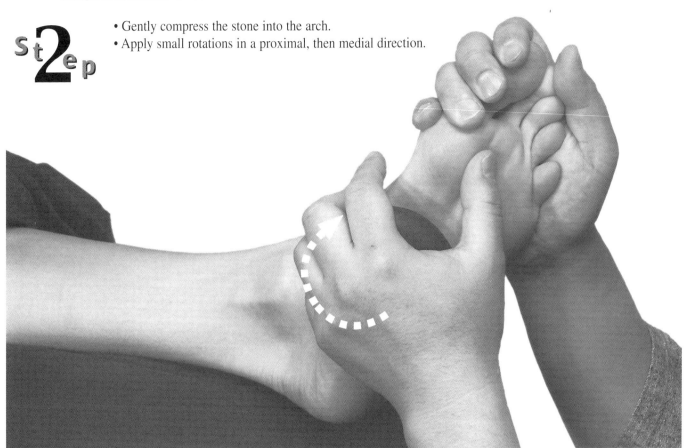

Step 3

- Move in a distal, then lateral direction to complete the rotation.
- Repeat five to seven rotations.
- Gradually reposition to cover the entire arch.

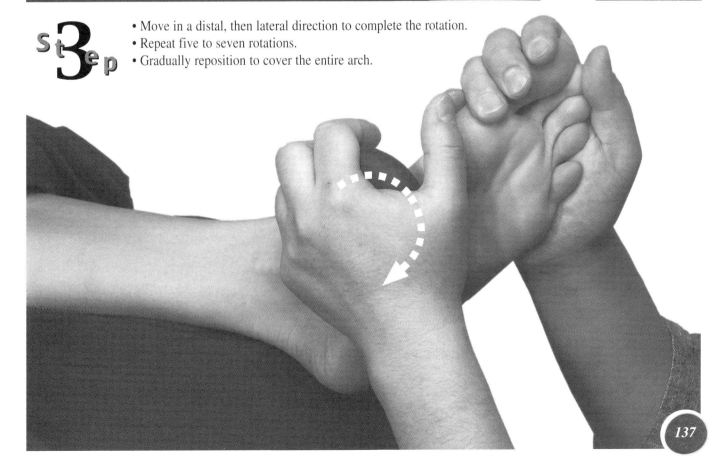

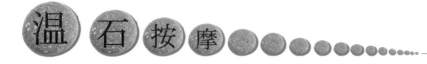

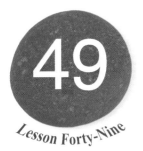

49

Lesson Forty-Nine

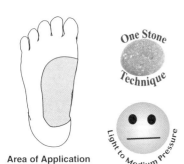

Area of Application

One Stone Technique

Light to Medium Pressure

温石揉捏法
Cross-Fiber Stroking on the Arch

This technique is used to deeply stimulate the arch. Releasing arch tension restores balance to the structural alignment of the feet, pelvis and entire body. With cross-fiber stroking, you grasp the stone like you would a chisel. Apply this technique with care, as the arch can be easily overstimulated. Asian bodywork is unique from most Western modalities, because it uses client body movement to apply techniques, rather than relying solely upon movement from the therapist's body. For example, this technique is applied by compressing the foot into the stone, rather than compressing the stone into the foot. Using body dynamics in this fashion ensures maximum therapeutic value with minimal effort, and reduces wear and tear on the therapist's muscles and joints.

St1ep

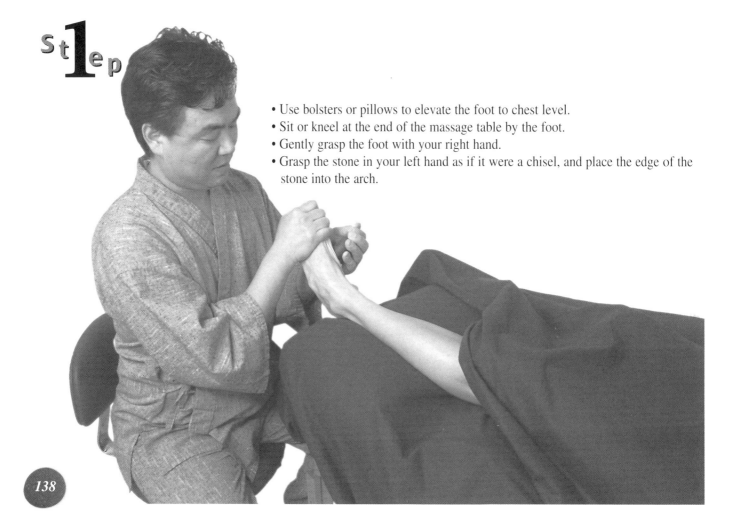

- Use bolsters or pillows to elevate the foot to chest level.
- Sit or kneel at the end of the massage table by the foot.
- Gently grasp the foot with your right hand.
- Grasp the stone in your left hand as if it were a chisel, and place the edge of the stone into the arch.

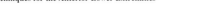
温石按摩

S t 2 e p

- Apply firm pressure into the arch with the stone.
- Do not hyperextend your wrist.

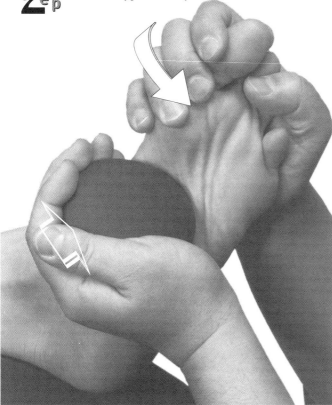

S t 3 e p

- Invert the foot to compress the arch into the stone.
- Repeat two or three times.

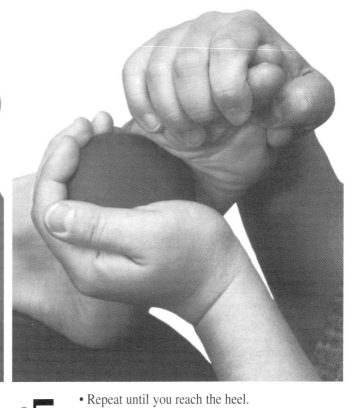

S t 4 e p

- Reposition inferiorly and repeat.

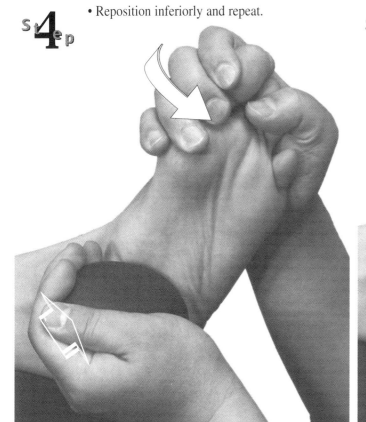

S t 5 e p

- Repeat until you reach the heel.

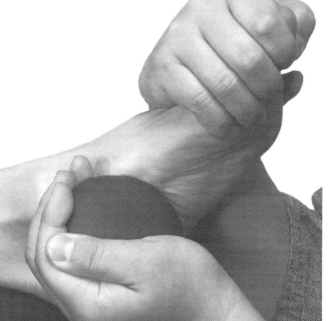

50

Lesson Fifty

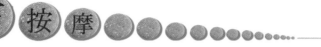

Rotation on Both Sides of the Heel

In Western reflexology, the lateral heel relates to the reproductive organs; whereas in Eastern reflexology, the lateral heel relates to the Bladder, and the medial heel relates to the Kidneys. In Asian physiology, the Bladder and Kidneys regulate the flow of liquid and fluid throughout the body. ("Liquids" being clear and white superficial fluids, such as lymph, and "fluids" being dense, thick liquid, such as the fluid in the mediastinum surrounding the internal organs.) Many tsubo in this area are very sensitive, so carefully rotate to remain within both a therapeutic range and the client's tolerance level. Do not slide over the skin while rotating; instead, engage and manipulate the underlying tissue. Keep the stone from contacting the malleolus or other bones. To smoothly apply this technique, use your fingertips as a pivot and allow the client's foot to move freely during rotation. Synchronizing your rotation with the natural rhythm and movement of the foot is essential for successfully applying this technique. Elevate the foot to chest level during this rotation. You should also face the foot directly, while keeping your shoulders dropped and your elbows tucked in, to maintain safe, effective wrist angles. When rotating over the plantar heel, slightly move your entire body to one side to maintain wrist alignment.

Area of Application

Two Stone Technique

Light to Medium Pressure

Step 1

• Use bolsters or pillows to elevate the foot to chest level.
• Sit or kneel at the end of the massage table by the foot.
• Position the stones on both sides of the heel.
• Adjust your body position to eliminate wrist stress.

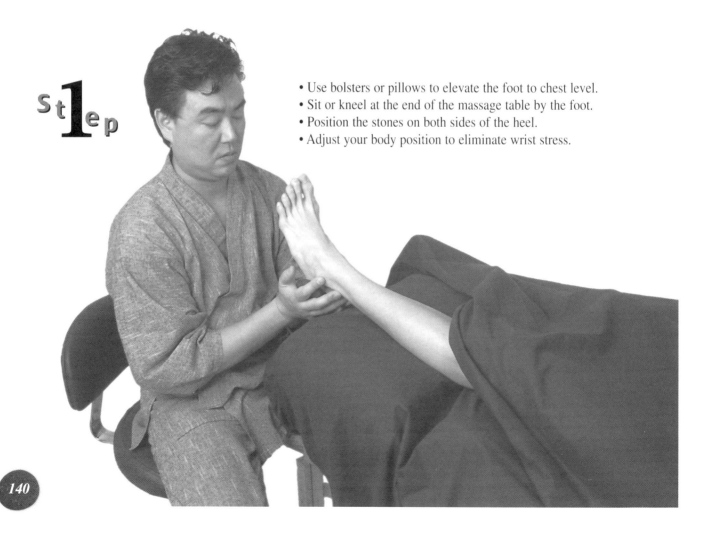

140

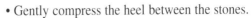

温石按摩

S^t2_{ep}

- Gently compress the heel between the stones.
- Apply small rotations with your right hand in a proximal, anterior, distal and posterior direction.
- Apply five to ten rotations.
- Do not slide the stones over the skin.

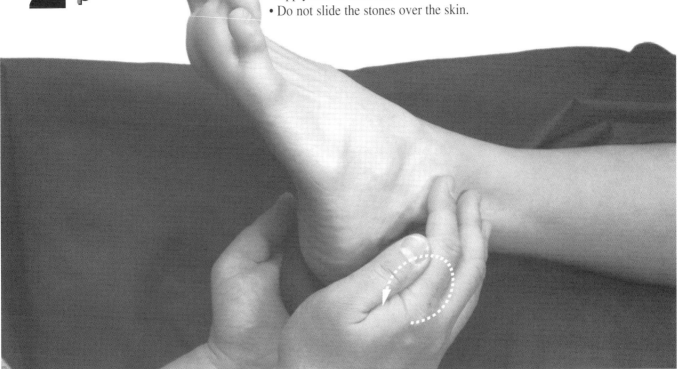

- Repeat the procedure with your left hand.
- Alternate between the left and right sides of the heel as desired.

S^t3_{ep}

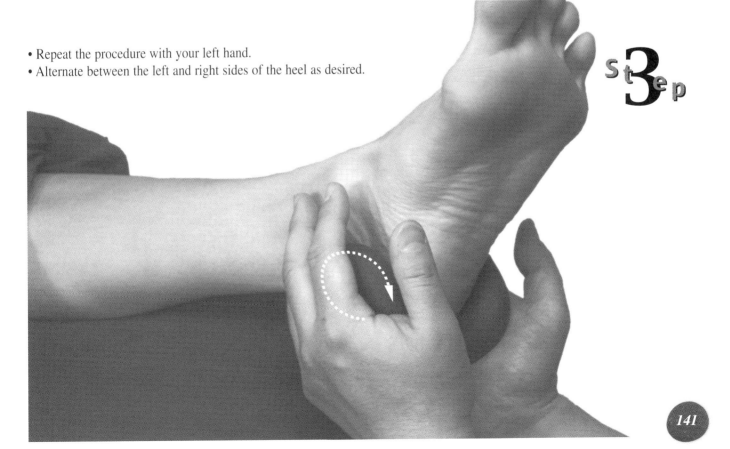

141

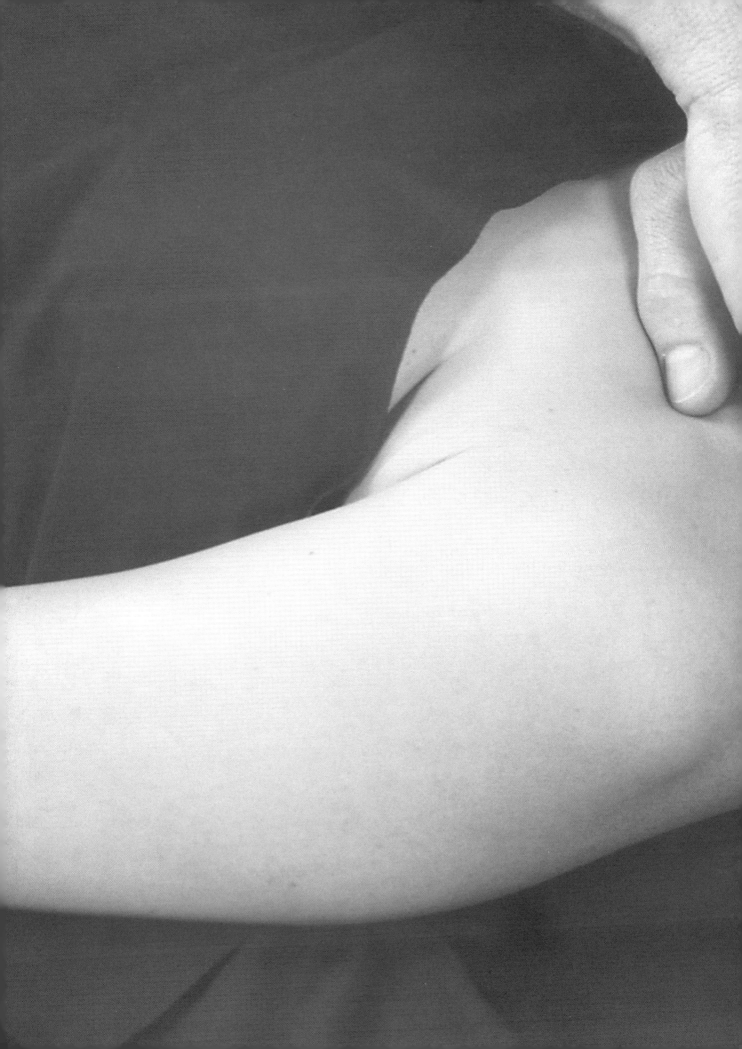

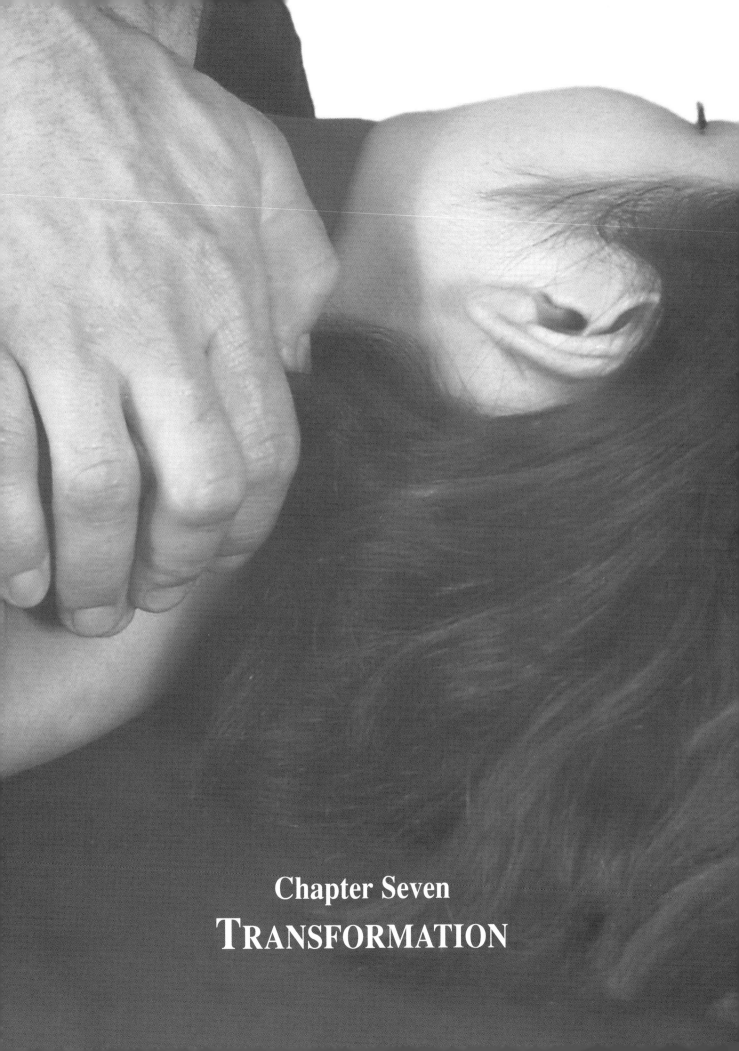

Chapter Seven
TRANSFORMATION

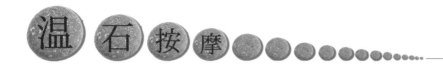

Chapter Seven
TRANSFORMATION
Techniques for Finishing the Treatment

This final chapter introduces five techniques to add a finishing touch to your treatment. This chapter also represents wood, the last stage of the five elements, that signifies growth, synthesis and transformation.

At this point, we have addressed the entire body with techniques from previous chapters. We now come full-circle to complete the treatment by working on the back. This series of techniques rebalances and fine-tunes overall body condition. The back, and the spine in particular, connect the entire body. Returning to the back at the end of the treatment transmits a message of finality throughout the body. These techniques restore the natural physical and energetic balance of the spine, central nervous system and entire body.

Both the beginning and end of a massage are extremely important. Communicating that the massage is coming to an end is essential for making the treatment feel complete. Your client should know the massage has come to an end without any verbal indication from you. The client should never feel like you've ended in the middle of a treatment. Their body should sense the end of treatment, and when the end finally comes, their body should feel deeply relaxed and interconnected.

This particular finish is vigorous, slightly aggressive and characteristically *yang*. If you prefer, you can also finish with calm, soothing *yin* techniques. You must consider many factors when deciding how to finish a treatment, including the client's body type, mood, health, and even the time of day.

Despite how you finish the session, the end of a massage is most memorable for the client and will, therefore, determine the overall quality and flavor of your entire massage. The end of your massage should be thorough and stimulating, but it should never cause pain or discomfort of any kind.

Unlike the techniques in the previous chapter which can be applied in any order, the finishing touch sequence should be applied in the order in which it is presented. This sequence will effectively rebalance the physical and energetic bodies.

温石按摩

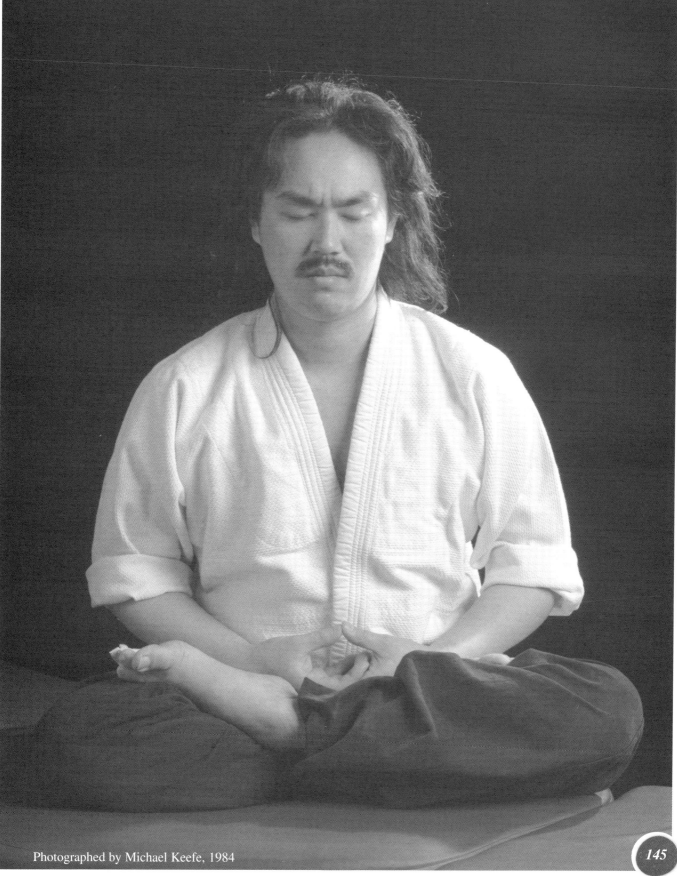

Photographed by Michael Keefe, 1984

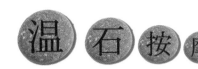

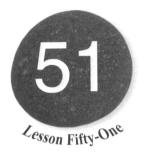

51

Lesson Fifty-One

温石軽擦法
Stroking Along the Bladder Meridian

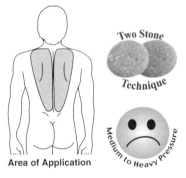

Area of Application

Two Stone Technique

Medium to Heavy Pressure

Finish your massage on the posterior torso to alleviate stress that may have developed during the session. Returning to this area also provides another opportunity to release areas that were previously adhered by compensatory tension. Begin the final series by stroking the Bladder meridian along the entire back. Begin with a fresh set of stones, applying long strokes over the Bladder meridian until the stones are cool enough for deeper work. At this point, the client is in a receptive state, so corrective and harmonious input will be most effective. The starting position of your stance is very important, because it enables you to stroke from the low back to the upper trapezius in one smooth movement. Keep your head and body posture upright when executing this stroke. The next few techniques are deep and slow, so acclimate each set of fresh stones with this stroking technique, before continuing the sequence. To deliver long, smooth strokes in a safe and effective manner, you must carefully adjust your body mechanics.

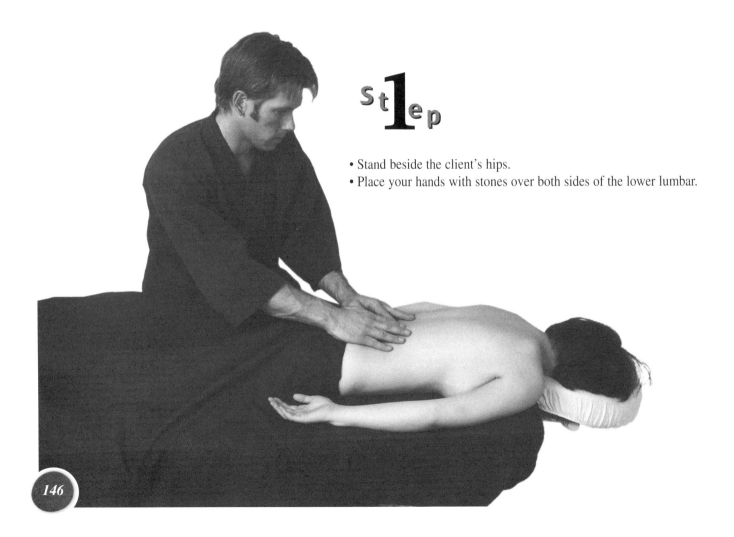

St**1**ep

• Stand beside the client's hips.
• Place your hands with stones over both sides of the lower lumbar.

温石按摩

• Stroke superiorly along the erector spinae.
• Do not contact the vertebrae, scapula or other bony surfaces with the stones.

St2ep

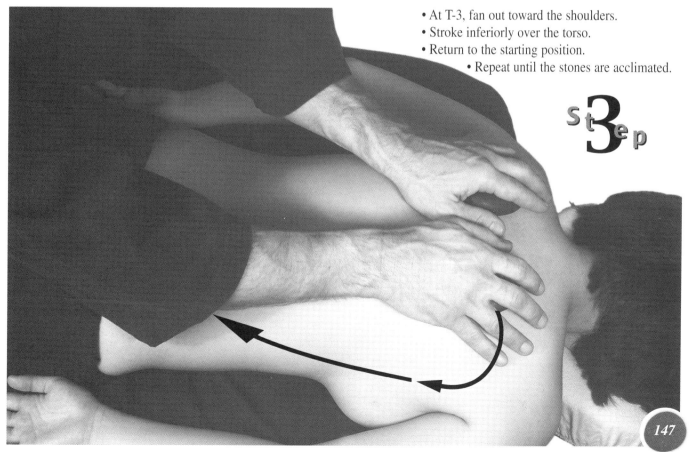

• At T-3, fan out toward the shoulders.
• Stroke inferiorly over the torso.
• Return to the starting position.
    • Repeat until the stones are acclimated.

St3ep

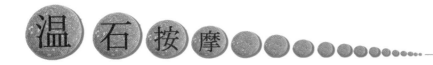

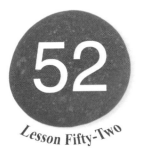

温石軽擦法
Deep Stroking on the Low Back

52

Lesson Fifty-Two

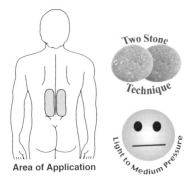

Area of Application

Two Stone Technique

Light to Medium Pressure

When the low back is warm from the previous technique, begin slow, deep strokes from the lumbar region to T-12. Apply this technique on both sides of the erectors. Properly execute this technique by sinking into the underlying tissue, while maintaining neutral wrist alignment. Initiate forward movement with your entire body only after you have engaged the tissue. When performing deep Japanese massage techniques, allow the client's *tao,* or body rhythm, to dictate the pace of the stroke. If you follow your client's lead, you will never go too deep. Check with your client to ensure they are comfortable with the pressure and temperature of the stones.

Hold the stones in your lower palm and push with your thenar eminence, not by gripping the stones in your fingers. Holding the stones in this manner provides optimal control while you stroke. Adjust your body mechanics by lowering your stance, dropping your shoulders and tucking your elbows to maintain safe and effective wrist angles.

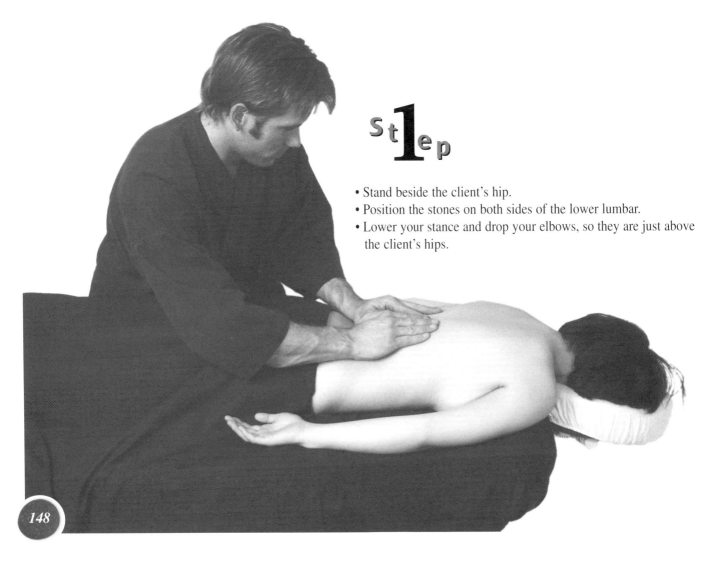

St1ep

- Stand beside the client's hip.
- Position the stones on both sides of the lower lumbar.
- Lower your stance and drop your elbows, so they are just above the client's hips.

温石按摩

Step 2

- Apply pressure with the heels of your hands to engage the underlying tissue.
- Glide superiorly through the tissue by moving your entire body.

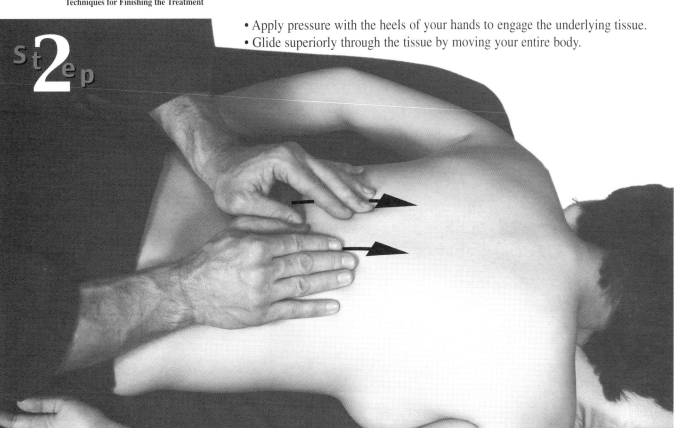

Step 3

- End the stroke at the floating ribs.
- Repeat two to three times as desired.

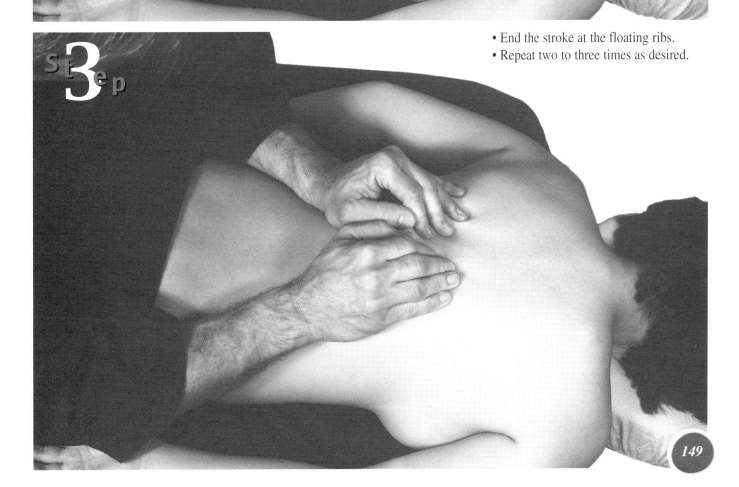

149

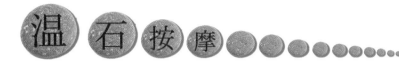

温石圧迫法
Alternating Pressure on the Thoracic Region

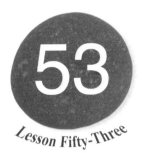

53
Lesson Fifty-Three

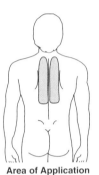
Area of Application

Two Stone Technique

Medium to Heavy Pressure

Alternating pressure along the thoracic vertebrae is the next step in this finishing touch sequence. Alternating pressure and walking down the thoracic region restores balance to the thoracic vertebrae. Carefully adjust the pressure during this technique to accommodate your client's sensitivity and muscle build. Adjusting your body mechanics is once again necessary to maintain safe and effective wrist angles. Lower your stance and drop your elbows, so they rest just above the client's hips. One alternating pressure application across the entire thoracic region is usually sufficient; however, you can repeat this application two to three times as desired.

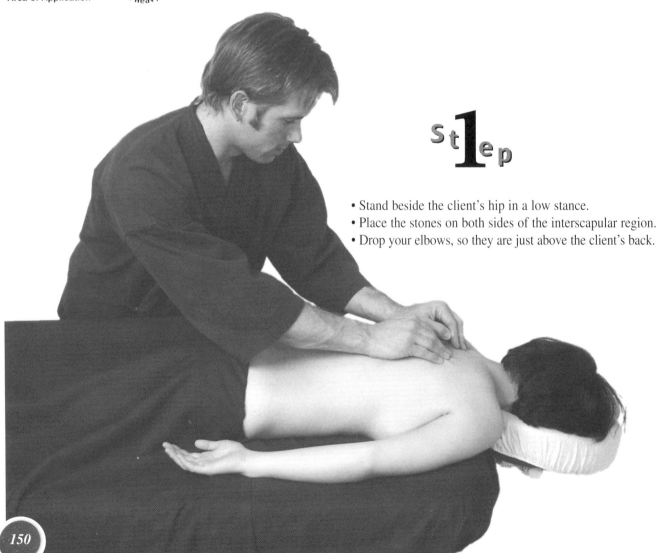

Step **1**

- Stand beside the client's hip in a low stance.
- Place the stones on both sides of the interscapular region.
- Drop your elbows, so they are just above the client's back.

Step 2

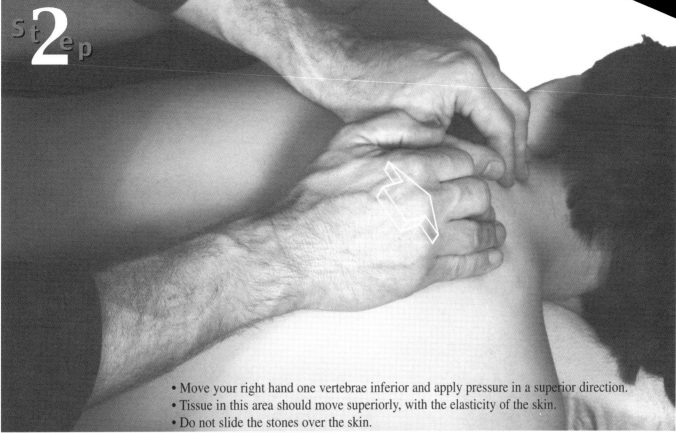

- Move your right hand one vertebrae inferior and apply pressure in a superior direction.
- Tissue in this area should move superiorly, with the elasticity of the skin.
- Do not slide the stones over the skin.

Step 3

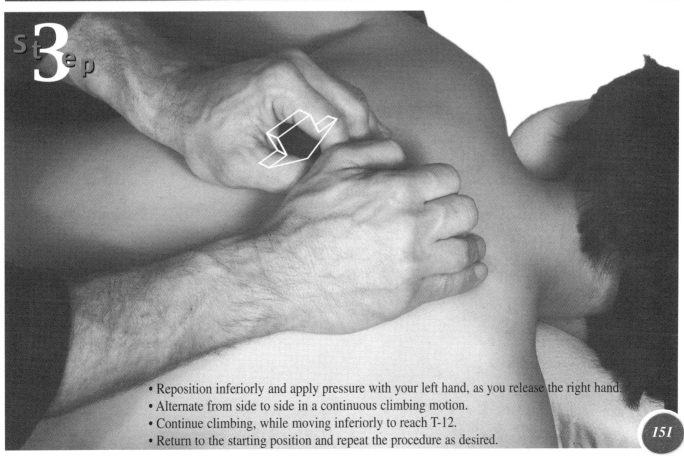

- Reposition inferiorly and apply pressure with your left hand, as you release the right hand.
- Alternate from side to side in a continuous climbing motion.
- Continue climbing, while moving inferiorly to reach T-12.
- Return to the starting position and repeat the procedure as desired.

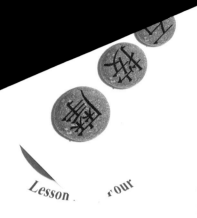

温石圧迫法

Inward Compression on the Low Back

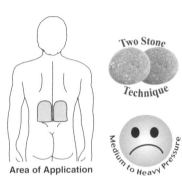

Lesson Four

Two Stone Technique

Medium to Heavy Pressure

Area of Application

Continue the finishing touch sequence with compression on the lumbar region. To apply even compression, equally balance your hands on both erectors, by extending your body over the table. This position has the potential to compromise your body position if done incorrectly, so proper body mechanics are crucial. Stabilize your stance by bracing your thighs firmly against the massage table, then rotate your torso into alignment with your client's body. Once you achieve a stable stance, you can apply this technique without any tension. Proper wrist alignment is especially important for this lesson. Do not lean your body weight onto the client, and keep your shoulders dropped and relaxed. The Kidneys can greatly benefit from heat, but do not overstimulate them. Kidney and adrenal stimulation, brought on by the effects of modern living, can be calmed by warmth and compression. To avoid overstimulating this area, pay attention to signals from your client, such as changes in breathing and audible sighs. This area is too sensitive to apply this technique with a fresh set of stones.

Step 1

- Stand beside the client's hip.
- Place your hands with stones on both sides of the lower lumbar, over the lateral edge of the erectors.
- Lower your stance to reduce wrist hyperextension.
- Lower your elbows and abduct them as necessary to maintain proper wrist alignment.

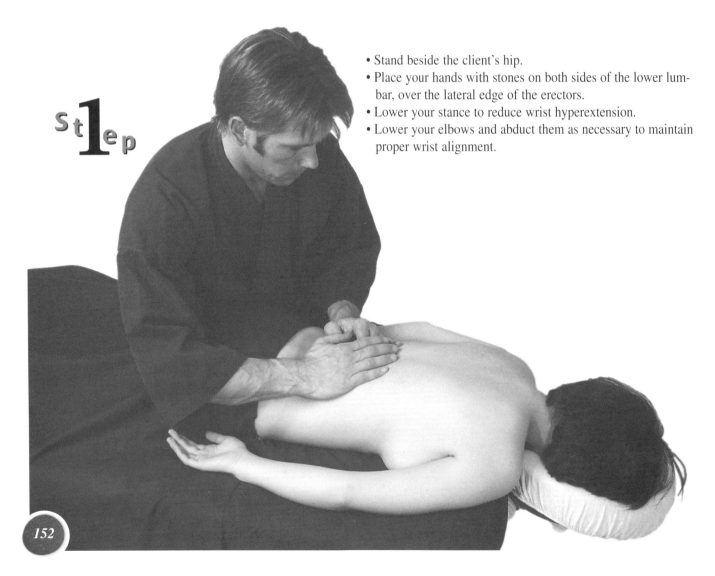

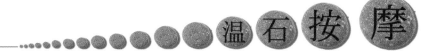

温石按摩

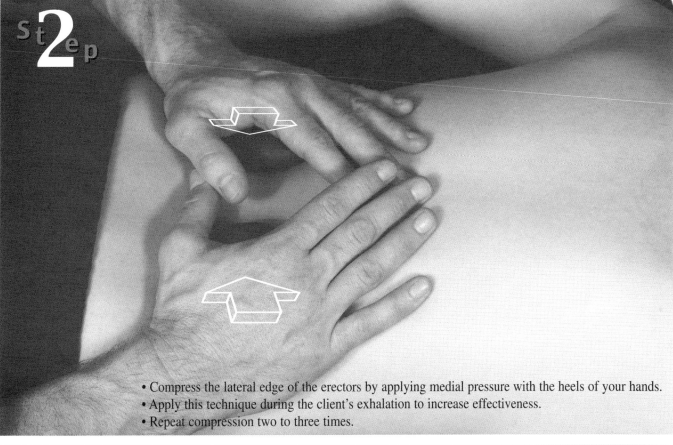

• Compress the lateral edge of the erectors by applying medial pressure with the heels of your hands.
• Apply this technique during the client's exhalation to increase effectiveness.
• Repeat compression two to three times.

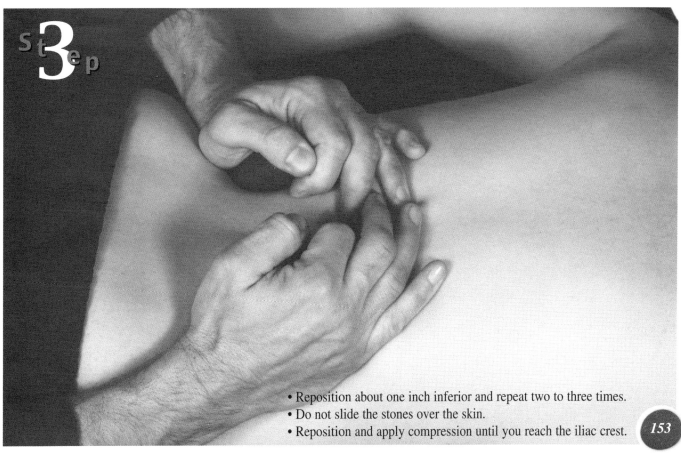

• Reposition about one inch inferior and repeat two to three times.
• Do not slide the stones over the skin.
• Reposition and apply compression until you reach the iliac crest.

153

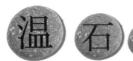 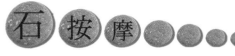

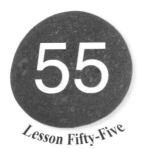

Lesson Fifty-Five

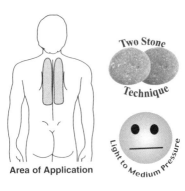

Area of Application

Two Stone Technique

Light to Medium Pressure

Compression on Both Sides of the Spine

This final stage of the finishing touch sequence gently compresses the erector muscles toward the spine. This technique is a common way to finish a Japanese massage. Compressing both erectors simultaneously allows the body to experience balance in these final stages. As you repeat this final stage, decrease the pressure to calm the client's nervous system, and suggest the end of treatment. As with the first touch, the closing touch brings the treatment full-circle and subconsciously suggests that the session has come to an end. Proper closure allows the body to accept the benefits of treatment and begin integrating them into the client's life.

Step 1

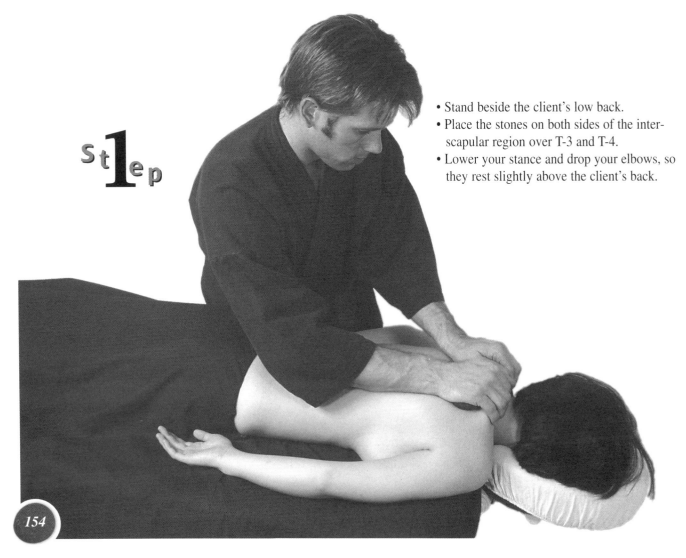

- Stand beside the client's low back.
- Place the stones on both sides of the inter-scapular region over T-3 and T-4.
- Lower your stance and drop your elbows, so they rest slightly above the client's back.

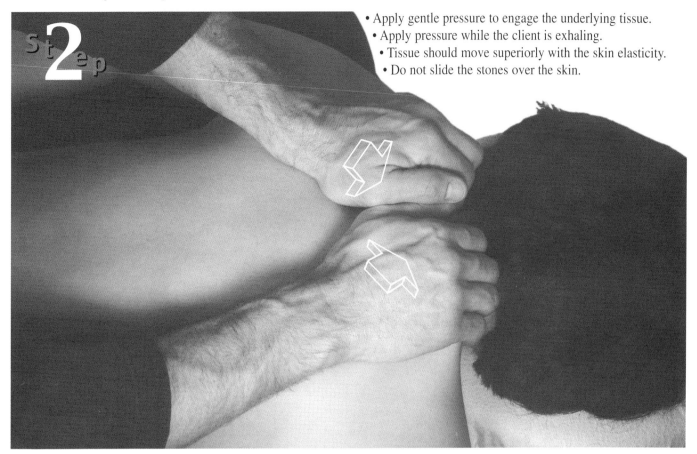

Step **2**

- Apply gentle pressure to engage the underlying tissue.
- Apply pressure while the client is exhaling.
- Tissue should move superiorly with the skin elasticity.
- Do not slide the stones over the skin.

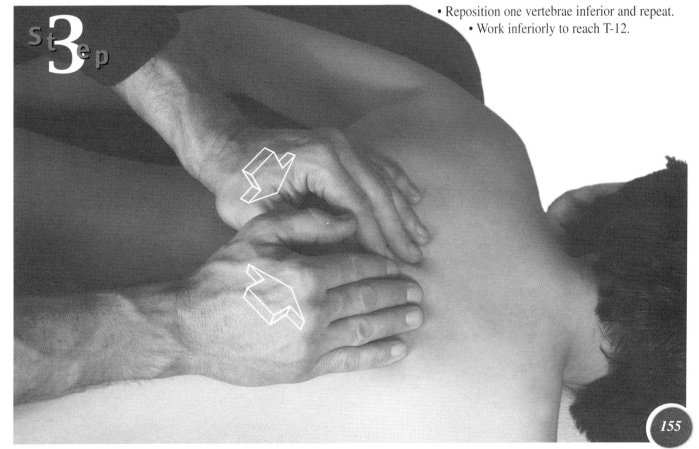

Step **3**

- Reposition one vertebrae inferior and repeat.
- Work inferiorly to reach T-12.

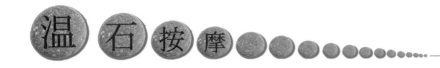

INDEX

BIBLIOGRAPHY

Anatomical References

Clemente, Carmine D. *Anatomy: A Regional Atlas of the Human Body.*
3d ed. Munich: Urban & Schwarzenberg, 1987.

About the Authors

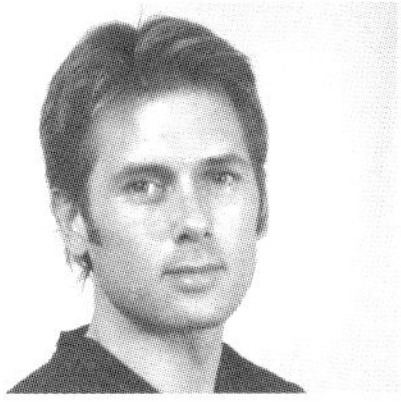

Mark Hess is a Licensed Massage Therapist and Instructor from New Mexico. He has taught at several massage schools throughout the southwestern United States, including the New Mexico Academy of Healing Arts. Mark's primary teaching emphasis is on proper body mechanics and hand maintenance techniques for students. He has extensively studied Japanese massage from Shogo Mochizuki. Mark is also a leading Massage Therapist and Spa Educator for the Ten Thousand Waves Japanese Health Spa in Santa Fe, New Mexico.

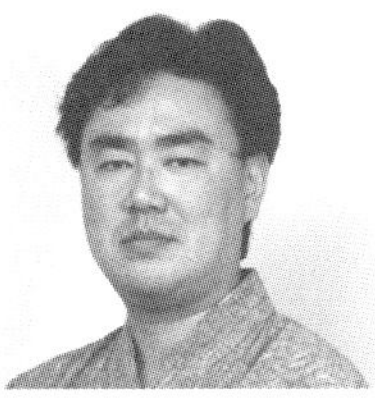

Shogo Mochizuki is a descendent from one of the most important lineages in Japanese medicine and massage. He has been licensed in Anma, Shiatsu and Massage since 1981 and has been practicing and teaching in the United States since 1985. Between being the Director of Education at the Japanese Massage and Bodywork Institute in Boulder, Colorado and a visiting faculty member at many massage schools, Shogo has taught massage and acupuncture to over 8,000 students in the U.S., Canada, Europe and northeast Asia. He is the author of over two dozen educational textbooks and videos on Japanese massage and traditional Japanese medicine, including *Anma: The Art of Japanese Massage*, *Ko bi do: Japanese Facial Massage* and the *Hand Maintenance Guide for Massage Therapists*.

Professional Training Books & Videos From Kotobuki Publications

Japanese Hot Stone Treatments

Japanese Hot Stone Massage

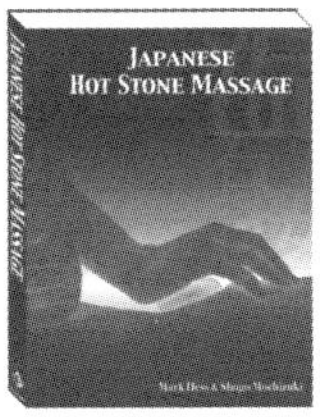

This book features:

- Japanese Hot Stone Massage application
- Easy to follow step by step instructions
- 55 techniques for the entire body
- Over 300 detailed photos and illustrations
- 155 pgs softcover, ISBN 1-57615-150-6
- $ 29.95 (Book only)

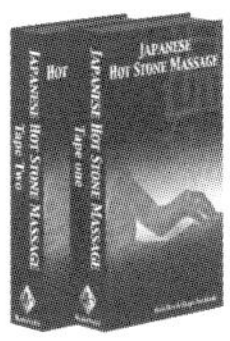

This two-video set features:

- Detailed demonstration of 55 techniques
- How to combine techniques for treatment
- Two 60-minute videos
- ISBN 1-57615-151-4
- $ 59.95 (Video Only)

Japanese Hot Stone Facial Massage

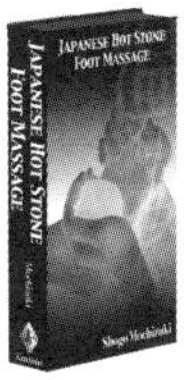

This video features:

- Detailed demonstration of 40 techniques
- How to combine techniques for treatment
- Approx. 70 minutes
- ISBN 1-57615-156-5
- $ 59.95 (Video Only)

Japanese Hot Stone Foot Massage

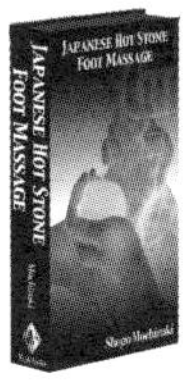

This video features:

- Detailed demonstration of 30 techniques
- How to combine techniques for treatment
- Approx. 60 minutes
- ISBN 1-57615-154-9
- $ 39.95 (Video Only)

Hand Maintenance Guide

Hand Maintenance Guide

For Massage Therapist

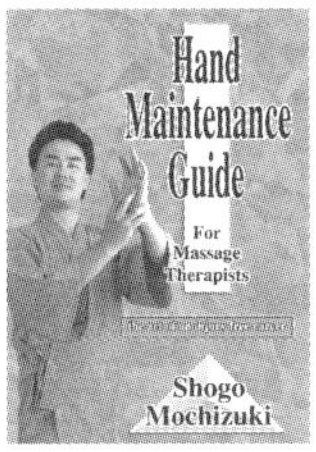

Hand Maintenance Guide Book Features:

- Why hand maintenance is necessary
- Causes of many problems
- 25 techniques for hand maintenance
- Over 170 detailed photos and illustrations
- 101 pgs softcover
- ISBN 1-57615-075-5

Book $ 19.95

#1 selling massage therapy injury prevention book. Required/recommended text for over 100 massage schools in the U.S.

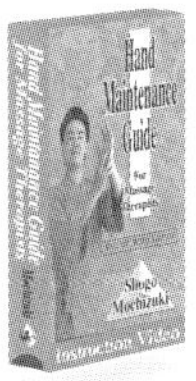

Hand Maintenance Guide

Instructional Video features:

- Demonstration on the causes of many problems
- Instruction of all 25 techniques for hand maintenance
- Approximately 60 minutes running time
- ISBN 1-57615-076-3

Instructional Video $ 39.95

To Order: 1-800-651-2662

303-442-6161-local/int'l

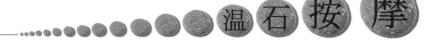

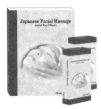
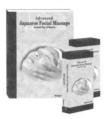
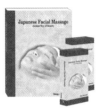

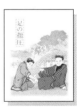

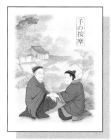
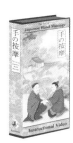
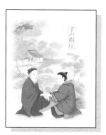
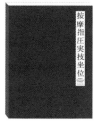
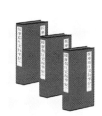
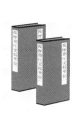
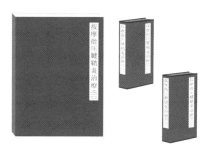

Workshops in Japanese Hot Stone Treatments

Japanese Hot Stone Massage

Two-Day Workshop

with Mark Hess & Shogo Mochizuki

Japanese Hot Stone Massage is one of the most therapeutic methods of massage. The techniques and theories are based upon traditional Japanese concepts dating back thousands of years. Unlike other types of stone massage, Japanese Hot Stone Massage is very rich in therapeutic value and can be applied in a light and gentle or deep and penetrating manner. Japanese Hot Stone Massage is unique, because it is not typically applied using oil or lubricants. These techniques can, however, be easily applied with lubrication for seamless incorporation into existing massage practices. Fifty-five techniques for the entire body will be featured, including passion, rejuvenation, balancing, calming and transformation techniques used to restore balance within the human body.

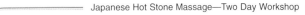

Japanese Hot Stone Massage—Two Day Workshop

- Step by step instruction of 55 Japanese Hot Stone Massage techniques
- You will learn how to give a full-body Japanese Hot Stone Massage
- You will be able to give light, soothing massages and deep, therapeutic treatments
- You will learn to apply Japanese Hot Stone Massage with and without lubricants
- Hand maintenance and proper body mechanics will be taught
- Instruction of Japanese concepts such as yin/yang, five elements, meridians and tsubo
- 90% of the workshop will be hands-on training
- No New Age ceremonial or unnecessary activities are included
- 15 hours of Hands-on Training, 15 C.E.U. credits and Training Certification

To Register: 1-877-651-2662

303-443-3434-local/int'l

visit www.japanesemassage.org

Shiatsu with Hot Stones

Two-Day Workshop

with Mark Hess & Shogo Mochizuki

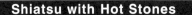

Although acupuncture dates back 7000 years, needle insertion did not begin until 2000 years ago. Before that, stones were often used to stimulate acupoints and meridians. Shiatsu with Hot Stones combines acupressure with warm stones to create heat therapy, such as moxabustion, while incorporating very slow, gentle movements and stretching techniques. Although this therapy is gentle and meditative, it is very effective in restoring peace and balance within the human body and mind. This soothing and rejuvenating therapeutic treatment is simple to follow and easily incorporated into practices, even for those who are not previously familiar with Asian bodywork concepts. This workshop is only offered two times per year and the Japanese Hot Stone Massage workshop is a prerequisite.

To Register: 1-877-651-2662

303-443-3434-local/int'l

visit www.japanesemassage.org